COMPUTED-TOMOGRAPHY A POWERFUL TOOL

FOR DIAGNOSIS OF PEDIATRIC AND ADULT CONGENITAL HEART DISEASE

METHODOLOGY AND INTERPRETATION GUIDE

First Edition

by

JAMI SHAKIBI, MD., FACC

MAHMOOD TEHRAI, MD., FSCCT,

AuthorHouse™
1663 Liberty Drive
Bloomington, IN 47403
www.authorhouse.com
Phone: 1 (800) 839-8640

Published by AuthorHouse 6/26/2015

ISBN: 978-1-5049-1427-7 (sc)
*   978-1-5049-1428-4 (e)*

Library of Congress Control Number: 2015909148

Print information available on the last page.

Any people depicted in stock imagery provided by Thinkstock are models, and such images are being used for illustrative purposes only. Certain stock imagery © Thinkstock.

This book is printed on acid-free paper.

Because of the dynamic nature of the Internet, any web addresses or links contained in this book may have changed since publication and may no longer be valid. The views expressed in this work are solely those of the author and do not necessarily reflect the views of the publisher, and the publisher hereby disclaims any responsibility for them.

authorHOUSE®

FOREWORD

New technological developments,in all branches of human endeavors should be approached with an open mind, developed and utilized to the best for the benefit of humankind.

Not all new developments live up to their initial claims, many so-called new developments fall in disuse or oblivion after a period of time. Computed tomography or CT-angiography has stood the test of time, in various branches of medicine, but in the field of congenital heart disease, pediatric or adult, it has a special place which has not been reported to this date in a comprehensive manner.

The author (JGS) has been actively involved in congential heart disease since 1970, and has grown with his patients, observing their problems during their growth from infancy,to childhood and adulthood. In contrast to the rosy days of 1970s and 1980s, as these patients grew older, the complications of the palliative and corrective procedures became apparent and the diagnosis and corrective procedures became more complicated, necessitating a great deal of effort to secure solid information before embarking on second, third or fourth operations.

The standard method to approach congenital heart defects for diagnosis and operative procedures was cardiac catheterization and angiocardiography, however over the years, and especially the adolescents and adults with congenital heart defects posed major problems, which necessitated a new branch of specialty, unfortunately disconnecting the continuous comprehensive approach to adults with congenital heart disease. This disconnection is most disappointing, both as far as the patient and the physician are concerned. To be able to render the best service to the patient, the care must be continuous and comprehensive.

CT angiography is a very powerful method to approach these complex cases, which could be used only by cooperation between an experienced specialist in congenital heart defects and a radiologist, well-versed in her/his specialty, who is interested in this type of patients. Thus this new methodology needs special endeavor on the part of two disciplines. This is in contrast to other fields of its use in which a radiologist could easily tackle the problem and report to the referring physician without needing a joint review of the case and a search for proper answers.

It is the authors' sincere wish that CT angiography be regarded as a major tool, besides cardiac catherization and angiocardiography in most cases, in initial and late evaluation of patients with congenital heart defects, especially the most complex cases, regardless of the patient's age.Of course cardiac catherization and angiocardiography especially when pressure measurements are needed remain as indispensable methods of investigation.

The authors are greatly indebted to Dr H. Emami,director of the executive council of Day Hospital for his invaluable support.

We are thankful to The Ethics Committee of The Day Hospital for permission to publish the data included in this book.

We are grateful to Mr Bahram Rimaz, Mr Masood Jahanfada and Ms Massuma Shams the super-technicians of CT-angiography Department of Day Hopital for their superb technical assistance.

The last but not the least we wish to thanks Ms MacVand for her secretarial assistance.

JGS and MT

Table of Contents

CHAPTER 1

BASIC TECHNICAL INFORMATION FOR CARDIOLOGIST USING CT ANGIOGRAPHY.

For technical, and theoretical information regarding computed tomography, and its application to the cardiovascular system ie CT angiocardiography major texts and references should be consulted (See Chapter 5: References). In this work we shall concerntrate on the method to diagnose congenital cardiovascular defects. However certain technical points are reviewed briefly.

Certain practical technical points are mentioned below:

1-The CT angios shown in this work were obtained by multidetector series computed tomography (MDCT). Data acquisition is spiral (helical) mode, 64-detector system are obtained per rotation.The manufacturerer is Siemens.

2-The contrast medium used for cardiovascular CT angio, is Iodixanol, trade name Visipaque. The dose used for infants and children is 1.5-2ml/kg given IV push.

3-If coronaries, root of the aorta, ventricular, atrial or cardiac valves have to be studied EKG-gated CT angios are obtained. However static organs like the aortic arch, pulmonary veins,pulmonary artery system etc, could be satisfactorily studied by non-EKG-gated image acquisition.

4-For infants an anesthesiologist versed in pediatric care is in attendance and Nesdonal or Ketalar is used for sedation. No medications are used to reduce the heart rate.

5- For studying fast-moving structures, ie coronaries, aortic root and ventricles EKG synchronization is necesssary.Thus for EKG-gated CT angiography, in adolescents and adults metoprolol is given 50-100 mg orally prior to the study. When the heart rate drops to the level of 60-65 beats/min data acquisition could be started.

6-For coronary artery disease,sublingual administration of nitroglycerin is recommended to improve visualization of the coronary arteries.

7-Arrhythmia artifacts, due to atrial fibrillation, premature ventricular or atrial contractions could be eliminated by synchronization with peak of R-waves, instead of RR-interval.

8- Some general remarks regarding **radiation dose.**

a-The radiation energy absorbed may be of various types: X rays, electron ie beta rays, neutrons, gamma rays,or other particles.

b-The radiation energy absorbed by the patient's tissue or organ is important, not the radiation generated by the equipment.

c-Therefore the **energy absorbed** must be divided by the mass of the matter. The energy is expressed in joules and mass in kilogram. In the international System of quantities and units, one joule /1kg is the special unit called "gray" (Gy) for absorbed X-ray.

Older units for absorbed radiation energy are:

1 Gy = 100 rad; 1mGy = 0.1 rad.

d-Radiation weighting factor or constant. This unit is a dimensionless unit used for reporting the magnitude of the biological effects of different types of radiation. The type of radiation used, affects the value of the radiation weighting factor or constant. **Radiation weighting factor or constant** shows the absorbed dose in Gy averaged over an equivalent dose (given in sievert ie Sv).

Thus this relation is expressed as:

equivalent dose (Sv) = absorbed dose in tissue (Gy)x radiation weighting factor.

The older equivalent dose (Sv) was given in **rem,** thus : 1 Sv = 100 rem; 1 mSv=0.1 rem.
As X-ray is used, in CT angio, the radiation weighting factor is equal to 1.0. Therefore in CT angiography, the absorbed dose in a tissue, in Gy, is equal to the equivalent dose Sv.

For Computed Tomography,other special dose quantities are used.These are:
1-Computed Tomography Dose Index (CTDI)
2-weighted CTDI (CTDIW)
3-volume CTDI (CTDIVOL)
4-multiple scan average dose (MSAD)
5-dose-length product(DLP)

The radiation dose received by the patient during cardiac,eg coronary artery study varies greatly depending on the type of equipment, EKG-gated and nongated studies.The radiation dose in one double-blind, multicenter report ranged between 568-1259 mGy x cm. This median dose-length product (DLP) was 885 mGy x cm.The dose received increases depending on the patient's weight, rhythm abnormalities and whether the study is EKG-gated or nongated .

See references under "Radiation dose".

CHAPTER 2

APROACH TO CONGENITAL HEART DEFECTS BY CT ANGIOGRAPHY

METHODOLOGY

Using CT angio for proper decision-making and to guide the surgeon for corrective or palliative procedures while dealing with congenital heart defects, is quite safe, easy and comprehensive. However to achieve this goal certain preconditions must be osbserved.

The cardiologist in charge must know the patient in depth and must have history, and physical examination findings in detail. EKG, chest-X-ray and echocardiographic data must be studied and recorded in detail. These informations must be used while discussing the case with the radiologist, and answers to major questions as delineated below should be sought with utmost attention.

When reading CT-angios the cardiologist and the radiologist must sit together, and while knowing the pathology, the radiologist finds the pathology and both physicians study the case in depth. Once through with the joint conference a comprehensive report is made which although including the CT-angio findings, but also giving an overall picture of the patient and the pathology concerned. **In this approach we report about the patient and the entire pathology concerned, not just a radiographic description of the images.**

In almost all cases, the data are quite adequate for surgical management. Of course when catherization is needed for essential problems, such as pressure gradients, ie direct pressure measurement, cardiac catheterization will be performed.

In this monograph,the approach to diagnosis of congenital heart disease is discussed in three sections:
1-Segmental approach to the definition of congenital heart defect.
2-Important negative findings.
3-Special pathology under examination, and final diagnosis .

Following these 3 steps, case studies of a wide variety of complex congenital heart defects regardless of age or parhology are presented.

STEP I: SEGMENTAL APROACH TO DIAGNOSIS OF CONGENITAL HEART DEFECTS.

To diagnose congenital heart defects, the authors use **the segmental approach proposed by van Praagh(1).**

In this approach one has to define situs first. Following that the position of three segments of the heart (atria,ventricles, and the great arteries) must be defined accurately.

Thus instead of using many confusing terms, the segmental approach allows a specific diagnosis of the cardiac segments, thus allowing a dynamic approach to diagnosis and surgical procedure.

See References under " Cardiac Malpositions".

1-DEFINITION OF THE SITUS AND VENO-ATRIAL LOCATION:

Situs of the heart could be determined by EKG,plain chest X-Ray, echocardiography and CT angio.

1-In **situs solitus** the liver is on the right side, the stomach bubble is on the left, and the heart is in the left hemithorax. **Inferior vena cava is right-sided and enters right atrium on the right side.**

2-In **situs inversus** the liver is on the left side, the stomach bubble is on the right, and the heart is in the right hemithorax. **Inferior vena cava is left-sided and enters right atrium on the left side.**

3-In **situs ambiguus** the position of these structures ie liver, stomach bubble and heart is indeterminate. Thus the heart or liver may be on the midline. **Inferior vena cava is on the midline and enters right atrium which is on the midline.**

Situs is mentioned first,ie:S= solitus; I=Inversus or A=Ambiguus.

What is most important, especially for surgical procedure, is the determination of **the venoatrial situs.** By this we have to determine where is inferior vena cava located. Once inferior vena cava situs is determined the atrium which is connected to it, is the right atrium.This is important for the surgeon. CT angio is a superb tool to show the inferior vena cava (which may be interrupted or absent) or the suprahepatic vein and the atrium into which it drains. **Thus by looking for venoatrial situs (inferior vena cava,right atrium) one can locate the situs as solitus, ie on the right, or inversus, ie inferior vena cava and right atrium on the left side of the spine or ambiguus, in which the inferior vena cava and right atrium are on the midline.**

CT angio frames showing venoatrial situs:

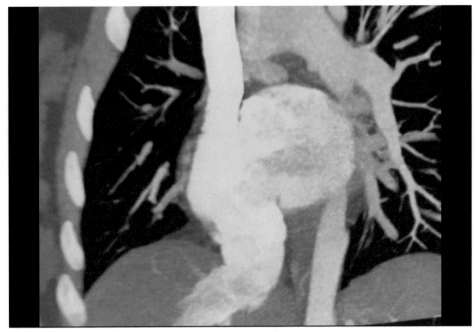

Figure 1: Visceroatrial situs solitus.Inferior vena cava and liver on the right side.
This means that right atrium is right sided.

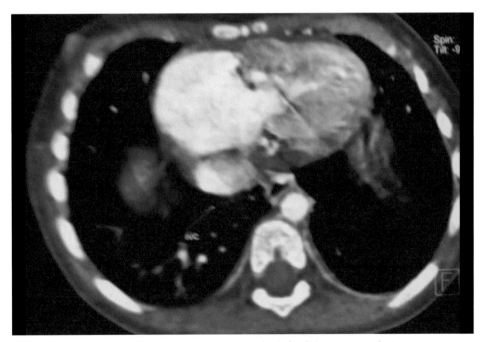

Figure 2: Situs solitus,Cross section,aorta to the left of the spine, inferior vena cava
more anterior to the right of the spine.

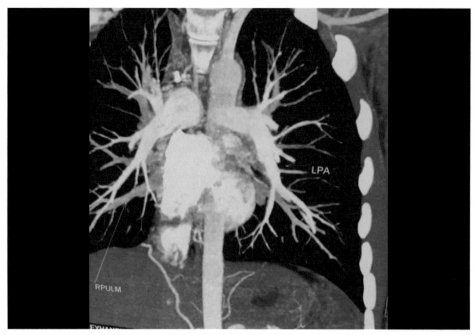

Figure 3: Situs solitus.Liver on the right, stomach bubble on the left. Heart on the right.

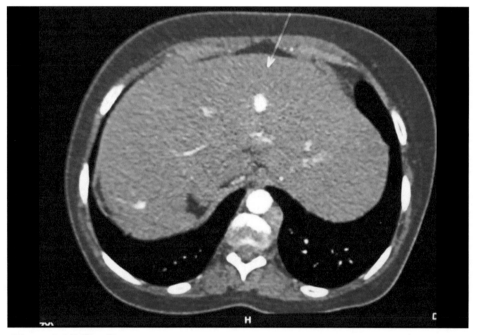

Figure 4: Midline liver

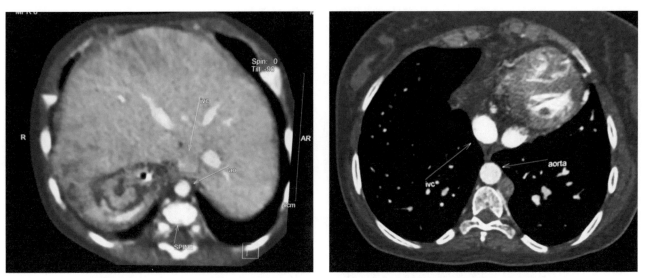

Figure 5: Situs ambiguus.Note inferior vena cava,aorta and liver in midline position.

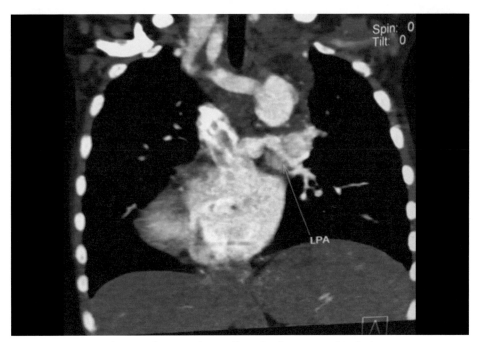

Figure 6: Situs ambiguus, liver in the midline, both aorta and inferior vena cava were left sided.Patient had right and left superior venae cavae.

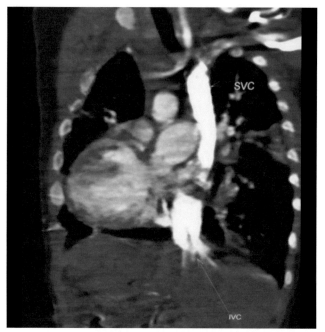

Figure 7: Situs inversus totalis .Note liver and inferior vena cava on the left and dextrocardia.

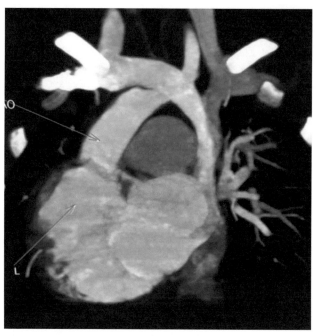

Figure 9: Situs inversus totalis, dextrocardia, aorta arising from the left ventricle.

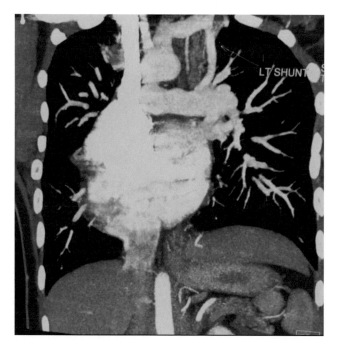

Figure 8: Dextrocardia with situs solitus, ie liver and inferior vena cava right-sided.

2-DEFINING THE POSITION OF THE VENTRICLES AND ATRIO-VENTRICULAR CONNECTION:

The physician who cooperates with the radiologist must use all the means, ie EKG,chest X-Ray and echocardiogram to define which ventricle is located on which side.Having this preliminary information one can use CT angio to refine the diagnosis. The important problem to solve is to define which ventricle (ie right or left ventricle) connects with which atrium (ie right or left atrium).Thus in normal state right atrium is connected to the right ventricle and left atrium is connected to the left ventricle.

Here it is important to use every possible method to identify the ventricles as right or left.

Specific criteria to diagnose the right ventricle:

1-Right ventricle is triangular in shape,in frontal view, with its tail accommodating the left ventricular body.

2-Right ventricle has a tricuspid valve.

3- Right ventricle has a conus which makes the outflow tract.

4- Right ventricle has a papillary muscle of the conus.

5-Inside the right ventricular cavity is heavily trabeculated.

6-Right ventricle has three papillary muscles.

7-Insertion of the medial cusp of the tricuspid valve on the ventricular septum is more caudad as compared to the medial cusp of the mitral valve.

Specific criteria to diagnose the left ventricle:

1-Left ventricle is conical in shape and rounded in cross section.

2- Left ventricle has a bicuspid atrioventricular valve.

3- Left ventricle has no conus and therefore no separate outflow tract.

4-Inside left ventricle is smooth.

5-Left ventricle has two papillary muscles.

6- Insertion of the medial cusp of the mitral valve on the ventricular septum is more cephalad as compared to the medial cusp of the tricuspid valve valve.

Not all of the criteria mentioned above, can be documented by any single method,except at autopsy or to some extent at the time of open heart surgery.One should use all possible means, to determine the location of the right ventricle and left ventricle in relation to each other (ie right or left side), and the atria. The physician who sits in conference with the radiologist to read CT angios must have done his homework to the extreme detail. In this regard, in a virgin heart one can use EKG for laterality of the ventricles. The rSr' in right the right precordial leads means that right ventricle (RV) is on the right side. In angiography during the catheterization one uses the shape of the ventricles (triangular for right ventricle in anteroposterior position and rounded for the left ventricle in anteroposterior position), the 2 papillary muscles in the left ventricle, smooth inside surface of the left ventricle and trabeculated inside for the right ventricle, could be easily seen and diagnosed.

Insertion of the medial cusps of the mitral and tricuspid valves on the ventricular septum could easily be examined on four-chamber view by echocardiography. However, one could see this also on special sections in CT angio. The ventricle under the valve leaflet more cephalad, is the left ventricle.

However in CT angio studies, using only selected frames, one has to be extremely careful, using these criteria for determining the laterality of the ventricles.

Although isolated inversion of the conus is described [See the second case described by JGS in epilogue], one can use conus for determining which chamber is the right ventricle.

For all practical purposes using CT angio only for determining the laterality of the ventricles, conus is the most reliable and easiest to see. So using CT angio, if the conus is seen the ventricle under this structure is the right ventricle and the ventricle which has no conus, is the left ventricle.

Using the papillary muscles, smooth or trabeculated endocardial surface, the general shape of the ventricles could all be misleading, unless supported by findings on EKG, echocardiography, cardiac catheterization, etc.

Once right and left ventricles are known one can describe the atrioventricular connection.Thus right atrium may be connected to the right ventricle or left ventricle and vice versa for the left atrium and the right and left ventricle.

By this stage one can say one is dealing with

SD;SL; ID,IL:or AD,AL;

SD means situs solitus, d-loop ventricles ie right ventricle is on the right and left ventricle is on the left.

SL means situs solitus right ventricle is on the left, left ventricle is on the right side.

AD means situs ambiguus, right ventricle is on the right and left ventricle is on the left, etc.

CT angio frames showing right and left ventricles:
As noted before left ventricle has no subarterial conus, whereas right ventricle is anatomically distinguished from left ventricle by having a subpulmonary conus.

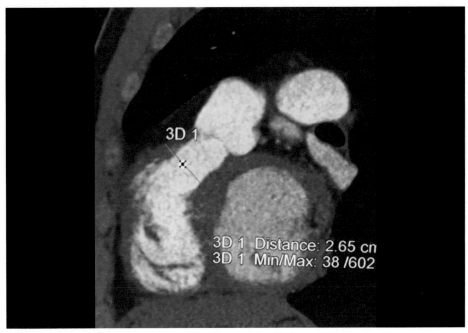

Figure 10: Note subpulmonary conus, a hallmark of right ventricle.

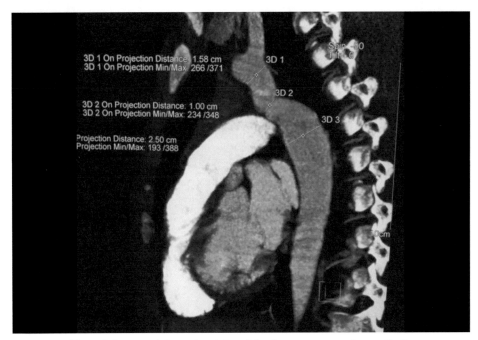

Figure 11: Note right ventricle to the right with a long conus underneath the pulmonic valve and pulmonary artery. Posterior to the right ventricle note left ventricle without a conus directly giving rise to the aorta.

Right ventricle is crescent shaped in axial section, triangular on longitudinal section or 3-dimensional view; and inside it is heavily trabeculated.

On cross section left ventricle is circular, whereas right ventricle is crescent shaped, covering left ventricle.

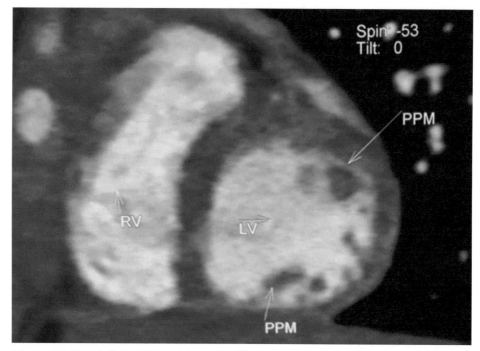

Figure 12: Note left ventricle with two papillary muscles.Right ventricle is crescent shaped on axial view cross-section, whereas left ventricle is circular.

This frame shows aorta originating from a heavily trabeculated ventricle, ie right ventricle .

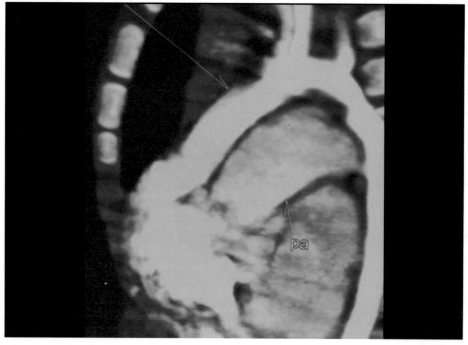

Figure 13: Aorta originating aneriorly from a heavily trabeculated ventrice, ie right ventricle.

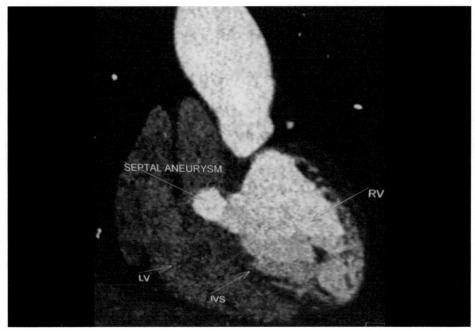

Figure 14: Note a heavily trabeculated right ventricle,on the left side. Aorta
originates from the anatomical right ventricle on the left side (LTGV ie
corrected transposition of the great vessels). Left ventricle is to the right.
In LTGV ventricular septum is perpendicular to the frontal plane, which
is in contrast to normal, in which ventricular septum is at 45 degrees to
the frontal plane.

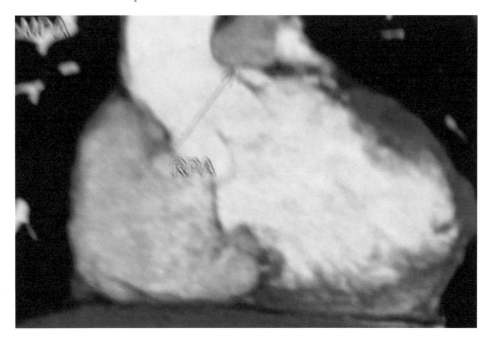

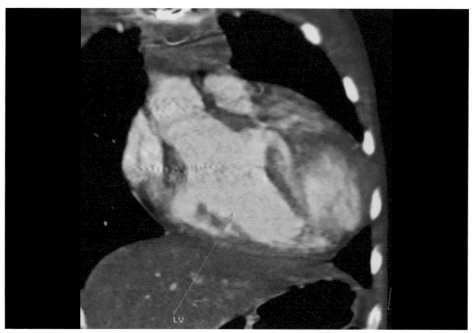

Figure 15: Left ventrricle is diagnosed by conical shape and 2 papillary muscles. Note the two negative rounded shadows on both sides of the left ventricle,ie papillary muscles.

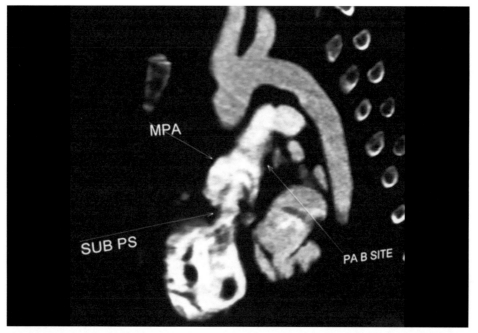

Figure 16: Note pulmonary artery originating from a smooth-walled left ventricle with two papillary muscles.Thus L-loop,LTGV(corrected transposition of the great vessels) is diagnosed.

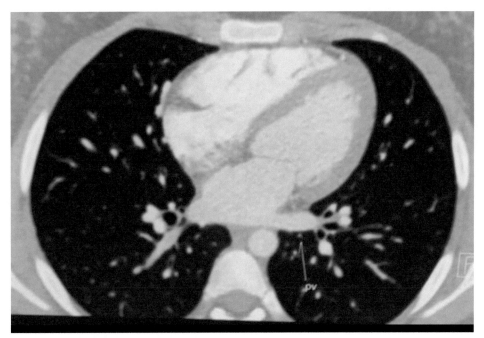

Figure 17: Right ventricle (top to the left) has a trabeculated inside. Left ventricle (top to the right) has a smooth inside. Also note left atrium and mitral valve connected to the left ventricle in front of the spine.

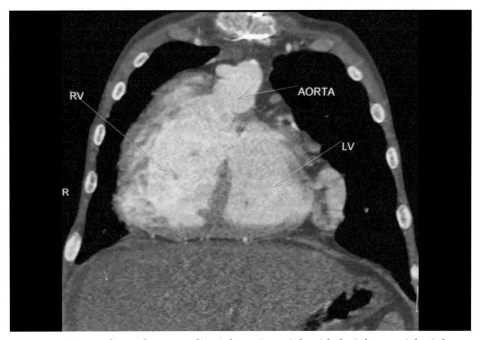

Figure 18: Situs solitus, dextrocardia,right atrium right-sided, right ventricle right-sided, aorta arising from the right ventricle, dTGV (d-transposition of the great vessels).SDD

For ventricles, if in situs solitus, right ventricle is on the right and left ventricle on the left, we have D-loop of the ventricles. So designation is given as:

SD;situs solitus D-loop ventricles
SL:situs solitus;L-loop ventrticles
ID:situs inversus ;D-loop ventricles
IL:situs inversus; L-loop ventricles.
AD:situs ambiguus; D-loop ventricles
AL:situs ambiguus; L-loop ventricles

3-DEFINING THE POSITION OF THE GREAT ARTERIES AND VENTRICULO-ARTERIAL CONNECTION:

At this step,the position of the great arteries must be defined. Thus one must give exact description of the aortic root and pulmonary valve location.

For each pulmonic valve and aortic valve one must define the position as right or left, anterior or posterior,superior or inferior. Thus in normal individuals :

The pulmonic valve is anterior superior to the left.
The aortic valve is posterior inferior to the right.
This is normal d-loop position.
If the **aortic valve** is anterior, superior to the left and
pulmonic valve is posterior, inferior to the right
we are dealing with **l-loop great vessels ie corrected transposition**.

CT angio frames showing the position of the great arteries:
Aortic and pulmonic valve position: d-loop,situs solitus. Normal.

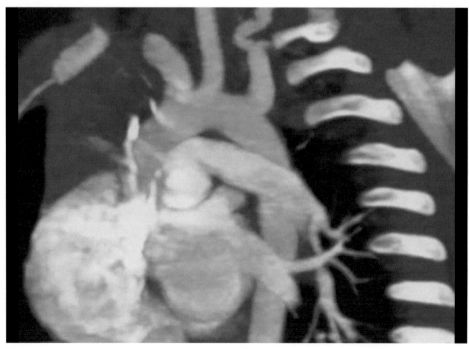

Figure 19: Normal d-loop position of the aortic valve and pulmonic valve.Aortic valve posterior,inferior to the right.Pulmonic valve anterior, superior to the left.

In the following case of a 3- month- old baby boy with d-TGV(d-transposition of the great vessels), aorta is anterior, superior to the right and pulmonic valve is posterior, inferior to the left, thus we are dealing with d-TGV. This frame showing the position of the aortic and pulmonic valves in full lateral position.

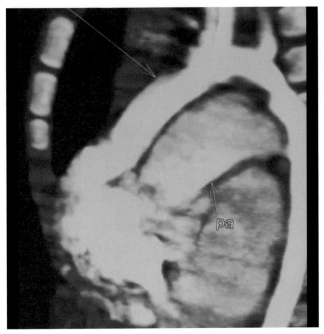

Figure 20: Figure 8:Aorta anterior and superior, pulmonary artery and pulmonic valve posterior, inferior,ie d- TGV in situs solitus.

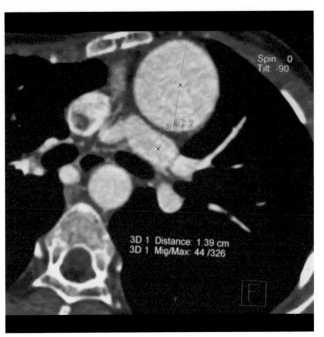

Figure 21: Inferior view, axial: Aorta to the left and pulmonary artery to the right of midline. LTGV(L-transposition of the great vessels.)

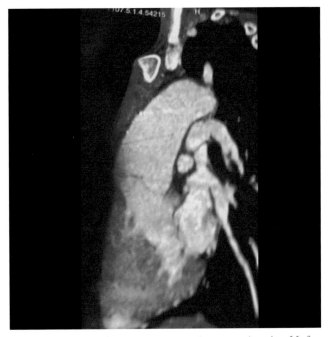

Figure 22: Sagittal view,aorta anterior,superior, (and left: not shown here) to the pulmonary artery, LTGV.

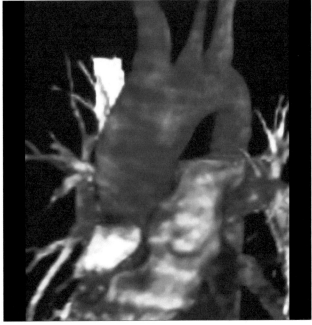

Figure 23: Aortic valve to the right of the pulmonic valve. d-loop.

Note d-TGV in a 2 month old baby boy with situs inversus and TGV.This patient has situs inversus totalis,with d-TGV. Pulmonary artery to the right and aorta to the left ie L-loop great vessels, so d-TGV for situs inversus.

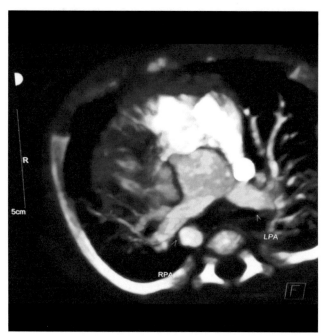

Figure 24: Situs inversus.Aorta to the left of main pulmonary artery at center,L-loop great vessels.Aorta orginating from anatomic right ventricle,next frame.

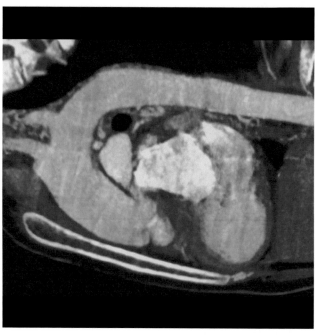

Figure 26: Note anterior aorta and posterior pulmonary artery with valvar and subvalvar pulmonary stenosis. Both great vessels originating from the right ventricle.

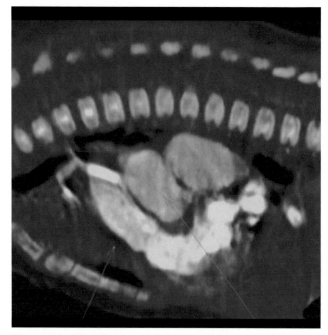

Figure 25: d-TGV ;aorta originating from the right ventricle and pulmonary artery from the left ventricle.

This frame belongs to a 17-year-old -female, with situs solitus, dextrocardia. This frame shows double outlet right ventricle.

The following CT-angio belongs to a 41-year-old man who presented with heart failure, obesity (101 Kg), who claimed to be unaware of his heart disease until 2 months prior to the outpatient department visit.

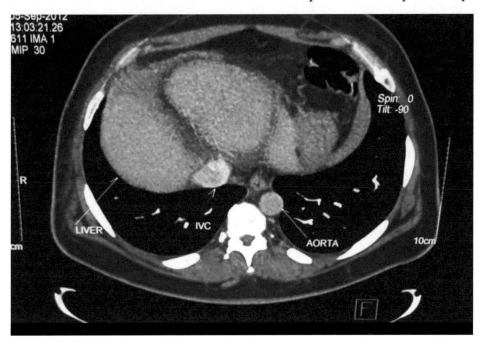

Figure 27: Aorta to the left, IVC (inferior vena cava) to the right, liver to the right, so Situs solitus.

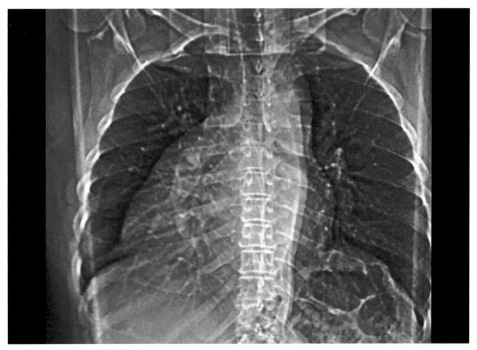

Figure 28: This CT-topogram shows dextrocardia, so considering the previous frame, this case is situs solitus, isolated dextrocardia,the heart can be to the right, left or midline. With these data RA(right atrium) is to the right and LA(left atrium) is to the left.The next step is to define the laterality of the ventricles and the great vessels.

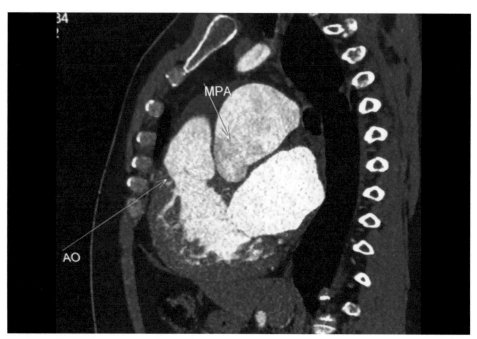

Figure 29: RV(right ventricle) with conus is anterior from which aorta arises. MPA(main pulmonary artery) is aneursymally dilated arising from the posterior left ventricle.

In normal individuals the great vessels are in d-loop position.

So to define the situs, ventricles and the great arteries, 3 letters are used:

eg:SDD, means situs solitus, D-loop ventricles, and 2nd D = d-loop great arteries ie aorta to the right (posterior and inferior), or if the 3rd letter is L, then it means, aorta to the left of the MPA (main pulmonary artery).

To practice, define these three cases:

SDD;ILL;ADD;

CHAPTER 3

STEP II: IMPORTANT NEGATIVE FINDINGS

Second step in reading CT-angios for congenital heart defects is to look for specific anomalies, which could be missed on physical examination, or echocardiography, and which could cause problems during surgery. Here a list of specific anomalies to be looked for is given.**It is important to report these items, even if normal, ie important negative findings.**

1-Is there one SVC (superior vena cava) or two ? One on the right and one on the left side?

Is IVC (inferior vena cava) present or interrupted?

See below under number 6 for figures.

2-Define the aortic arch, as far as laterality (right or left), shape and diameter in various segments is concerned. Specifically aortic isthmus should be evaluated carefully.

3-While studying aortic arch specific mention must be made regarding coarctation of the aorta and PDA(patent ductus arteriosus).

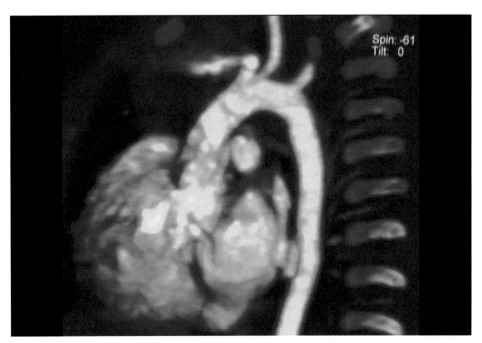

Figure 30: Normal aortic arch. No PDA (patent ductus arteriosus),no coarctation of the aorta.

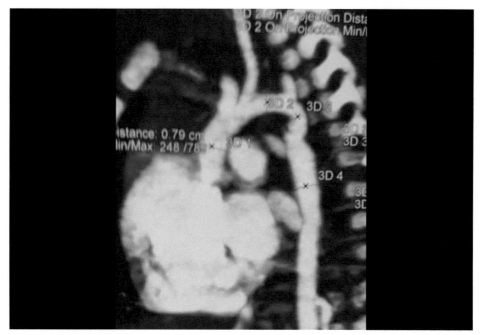

Figure 31: Normal aortic arch.

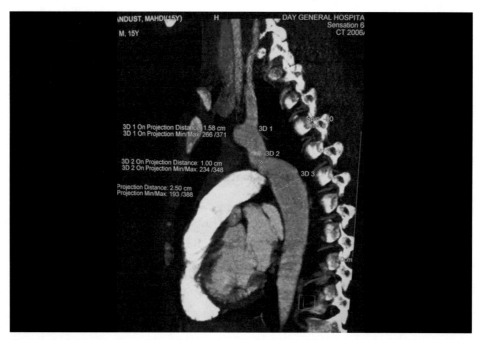

Figure 32: Note incidental finding of a cervical aorta, with tortuous isthmus and mild coarctation of the aorta in a 15-year-old male with Marfan's syndrome and polyvalvar dysplasia.

Aortic arch is embryologically derived from the 4th branchial arch. As the origin and embryogenesis of this structure is very complex, it is usually of different shapes and diameters in its ascending, transverse and descending parts. Note the different shapes and diameters in the above figure, from a 2-month-old baby girl who had TAPVD(total anomalous pulmonary venous drainage). Special care should be exercised while studying the aortic arch and its major branches.Absence of anomalies such as coarctation and PDA(patent ductus arteriosus) must be reported as important negative findings.

4-On which side is the descending aorta?

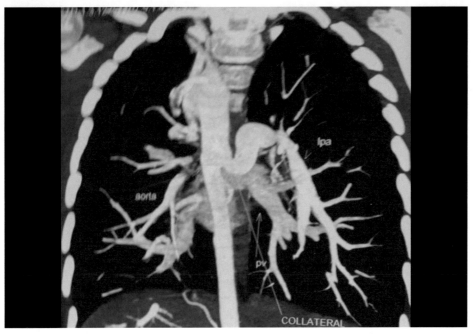

Figure 33: Note right aortic arch and descending aorta. Also a large left collateral
artery feeding the left lung.

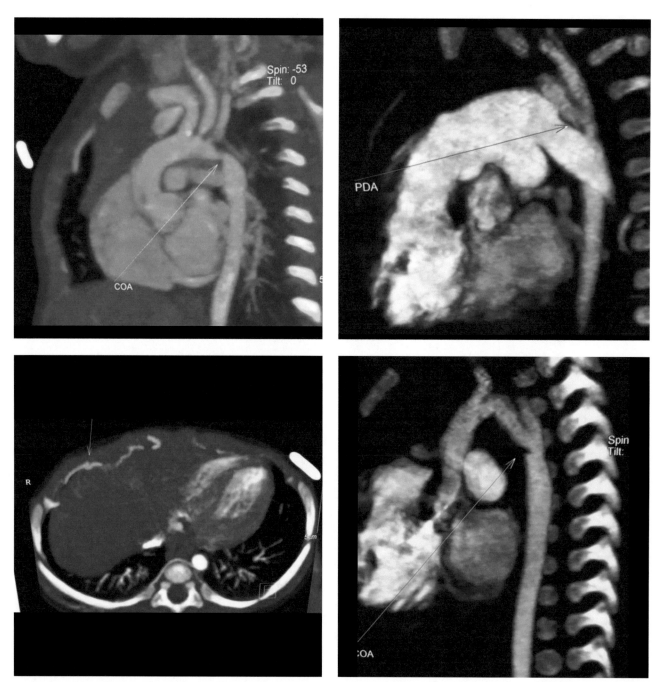

Figure 34: Discrete CoA (coarctation of the aorta) with collaterals (bottom frame, arrow).

Figure 35: PDA (patent ductus arteriosus) (top frame) and juxtaductal coarctation of the aorta (bottom frame) in a 3-month-old girl with large VSD (ventricular septal defect).

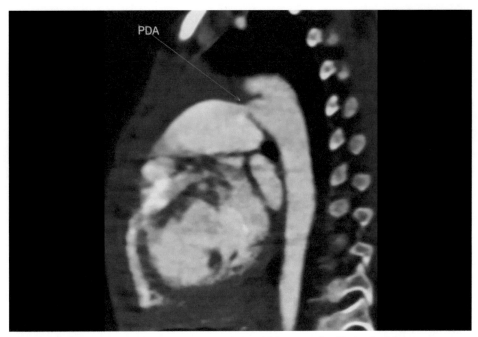

Figure 36: PDA (patent ductus arteriosus)should be specifically looked for.

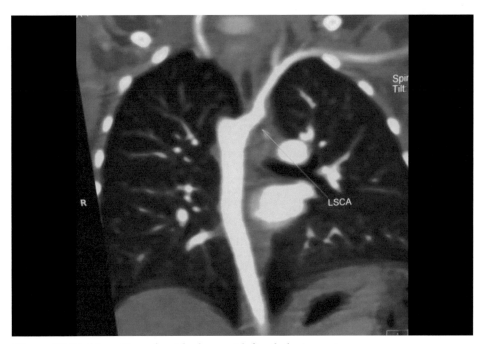

Figure 37: Right aortic arch with aberrant left subclavian artery.

5-Look for the coronaries, and make sure there are two ostia and proximal segments are normal.

Although CT angio for coronary artery disease, is a separate field of study, the physician dealing with congenital heart disease cannot ignore coronary arteries. One must look for anomalies of the coronary arteries, noted in many congenital heart defects, such as TF (tetralogy of Fallot),L-TGV (L transposition of the great arteries), etc. The physician must be familiar with the normal coronary artery anatomy.It is important to add a note to the final interpretation of the frames, regarding the state of the coronaries. Normal coronaries is an important negative finding to be reported for most anomalies under study. Also for older patients who go for repeat operations, for their congenital heart defects,the report must include detailed study of their coronaries.

Because of the importance of the coronary arteries, a short review of the normal coronaries is given below. (For references look under "Coronary arteries".)

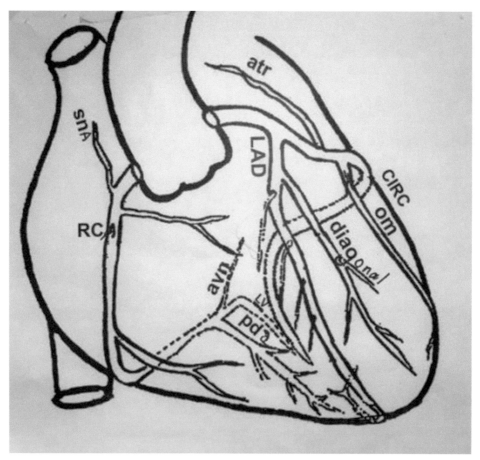

Figure 38: Schematic drawing of the normal coronaries and branches.

Left main coronary artery arises above the left coronary cusp of the aorta, and it gives rise to LAD (left anteriror descending) and CX (circumflex) branches.OM (obtuse marginal) and diagonal branches originate from the CX and LAD respectively. RCA(right coronary artery) originates above the right coronary cusp of the aorta and gives AVN (atrioventricualar nodal) and PD (posterior descending) branches. Terminal branches of the CX, LAD and RCA feed the ventricular myocardium.

Normal coronaries are shown below on CT angio VRT images. Using the above diagram, identify the branches shown. The patient is a 30-year old-male being considered for repair of his RVOT (right ventricular outflow tract) patch and pulmonic valve replacement.The coronaries were normal.

(1)-Anterior frontal right

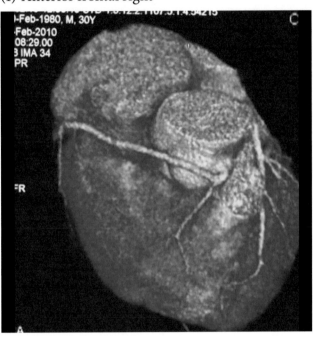

(3)-Anterior right frontal

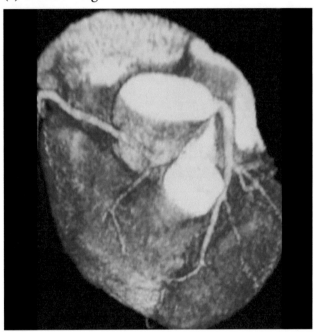

(2)-Anterior horizontal left.

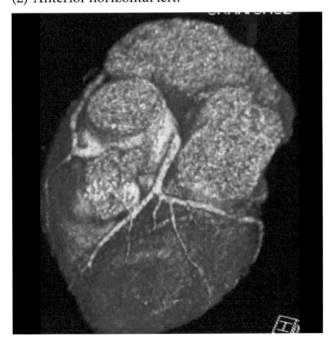

(4)-Frontal right posterior

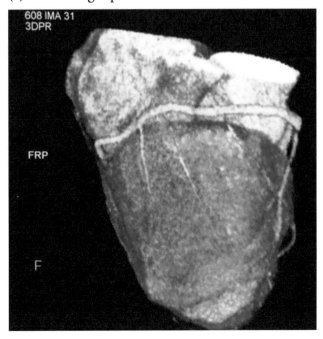

(5)-Posterior frontal left

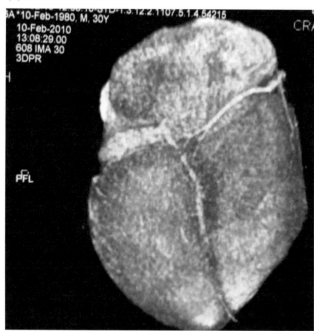

(7)- Horizontal anterior right.

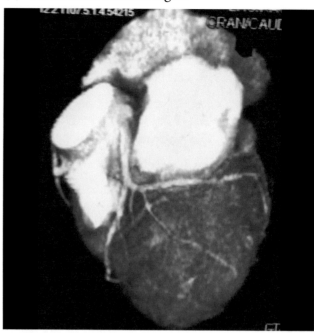

(6)-Anterior right frontal

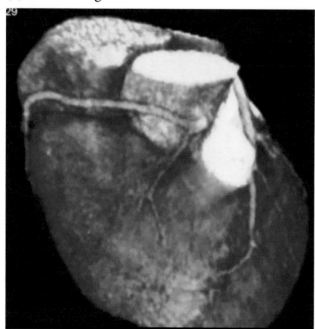

(8)- Posterior left frontal

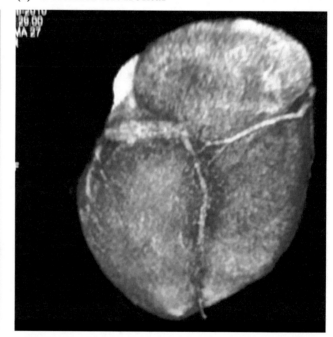

(9)-Front right posterior

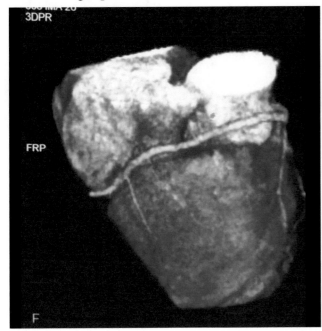

(11)-Right posterior frontal

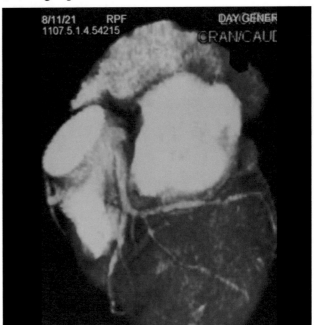

(10)-Anterior front right

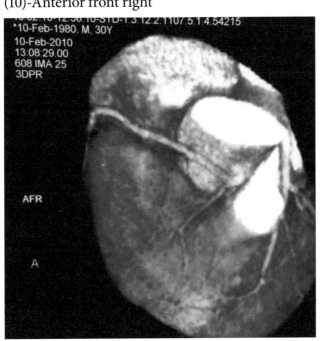

These frames belong to a 38-year-old male with normal coronary arteries.

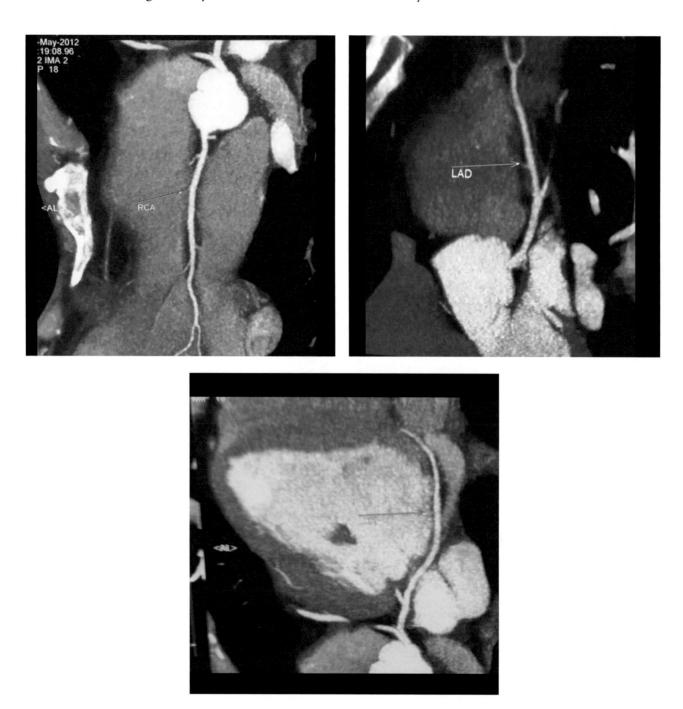

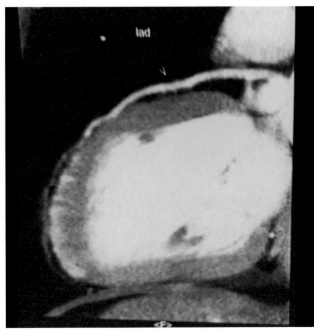

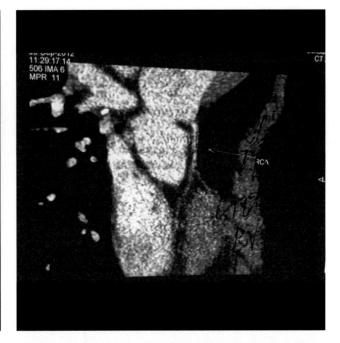

Figure 39: These frames belong to a 38-year-old male with normal coronary arteries.Top to bottom: RCA(right coronary artery),LCX(left circumflex),LAD(left anterior descending).

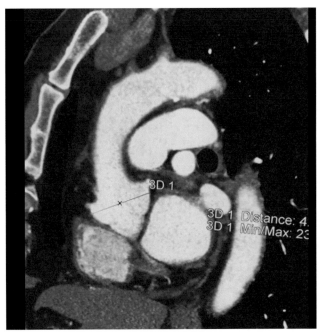

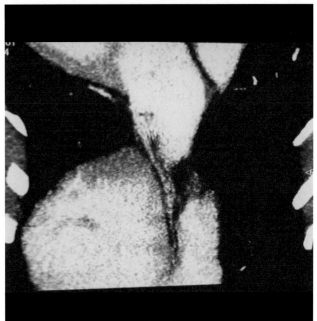

Figure 41: Patient with tetralogy of Fallot, acquired pulmonary atresia. Top frame shows LAD(left anterior descending) arising from RCA (right coronary artery), and bottom frame showing LAD crossing in front of the RVOT(right ventricular outflow tract).

Figure 40: Isolated aneurysmal dilation of the sinus of Valsalva, 4.39 cm in diameter, in a 65-year-old male with 2 stents.

Continuing "important negative findings."

6-Is there a left SVC (superior vena cava)? If so report its drainage site.

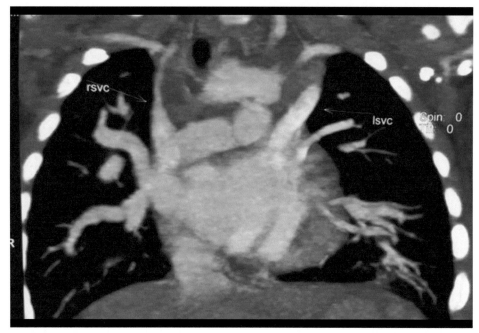

Figure 42: SVC draining into the RA (right atrim). Also note IVC (inferior vena cava).
On the left, there is a left SVC draining into the coronary sinus.

7-Look at all 4 pulmonary veins and make specific report about the drainage of all veins into the left atrium.

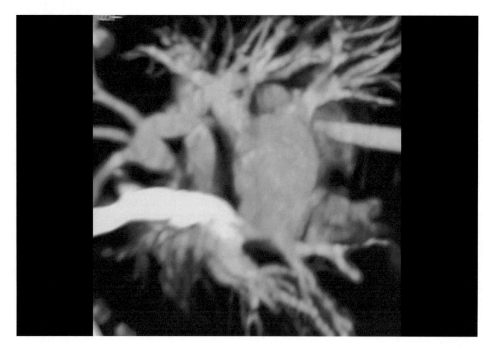

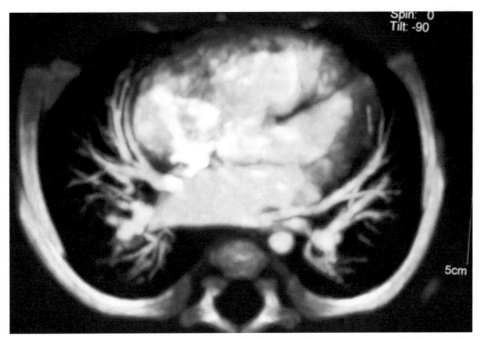

Figure 43: All four pulmonary veins must be shown to drain into the LA (left atrium), the Crab sign.

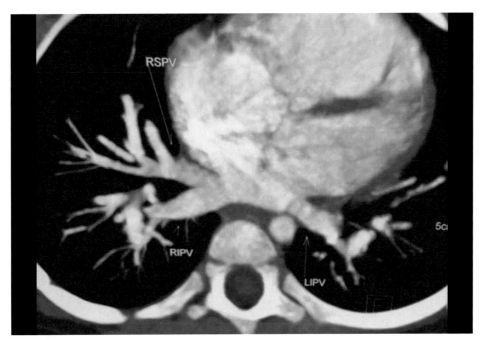

Figure 44: In all atrial septal defects regardless of the type it is mandatory to identify all four pulmonary veins and their drainage site. Partial anomalous pulmonary venous return could be a great nuisance,if undetected and found at the time of surgery.This figure shows normal pulmonary venous return.

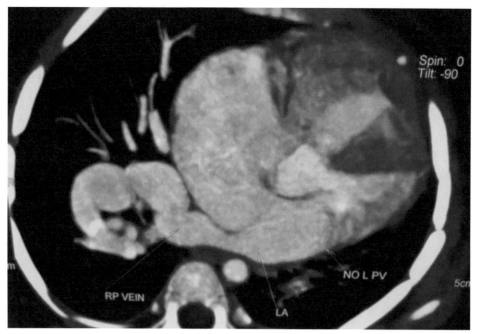

Figure 45: Note aneurysmal right pulmonary veins and agenesis of the left pulmonary veins.

The following two frames show TAPVD (total anomalous pulmonary venous drainage) into the low SVC(superior v ena cava), in a 4 -year-old boy with Ivemark syndrome, DORV(double outlet right ventricle) and hypoplastic MV(mitral valve) and LV(left ventricle).

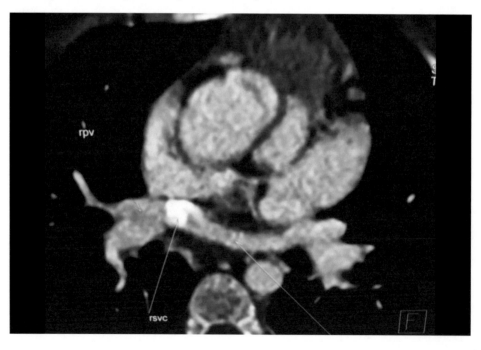

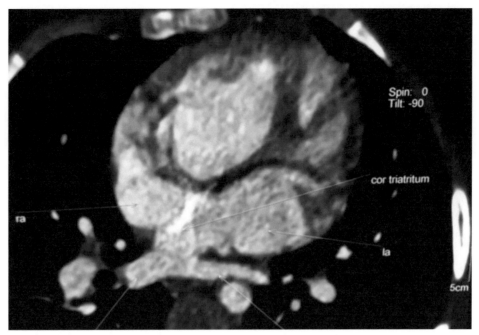

Figure 46: Right and left pulmonary veins drain into low right SVC(superior vena cava).

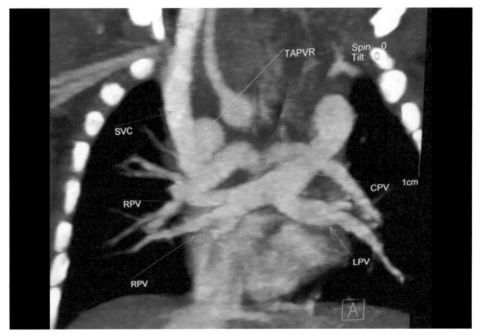

Figure 47: TAPVD into low SVC.

8-Regarding the pulmonary artery, mention confluency of the MPA(main pulmonary artery),LPA and RPA (left and right pulmonary arteries). Report the general size and development of the major branches and presence of collaterals if any.

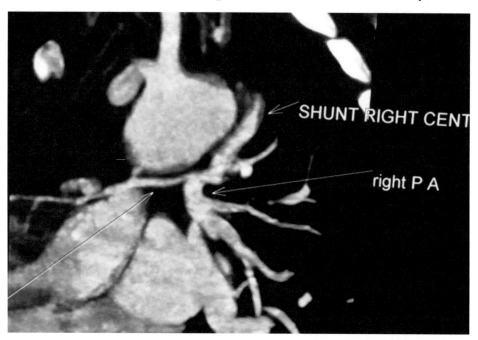

Figure 48: Posterior view. Hypoplastic RPA (right pulmonary artery) fed by a right central shunt. Unmarked arrow on the left shows a hypoplastic MPA(main pulmonary artery) with pulmonary atresia, continuing into a thread-like LPA(left pulmonary artery).

In the following two frames note that this 50-day-old boy with large perimembranous VSD (ventricular septal defect), and severe pulmonary hypertension, had confluent pulmonary artery with normal anatomy (top frame). Following PA banding at the age of 20 months, pulmonary artery band has migrated to the distal MPA(main pulmonary artery) causing severe stenosis (bottom frame).

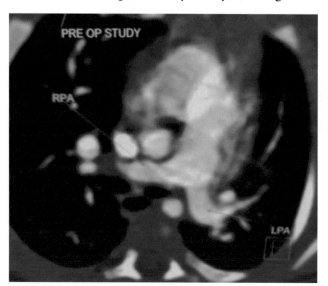
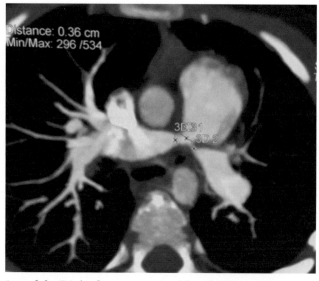

Figure 49: At 20 months of age,this study shows distal migration of the PA (pulmonary artery) band.MPA(main pulmonart artery) 0.45 cm, LPA(left pulmonary artery) origin 0.19 cm,RPA (right pulmonary artery) origin o.36 cm in diameter.

CHAPTER 4

STEP III: SPECIFIC ANOMALIES. CASE STUDIES

References are given under specific diagnoses in the section of "References".

Case study:MM #001

Patient is a 23-year-old girl followed since 21 months of age. The patient is erratic in follow-up visits and consults several physicians simultaneously. She had tricuspid atresia type IA. Pulmonary artery system was hypoplastic with bilateral left and right pulmonary artery origin stenosis. Because of severe cyanosis she underwent a left Goretex shunt at 5 years of age.

At 7 years of age, left pulmonary artery measured 7 mm in diameter and right pulmonary artery was 12 mm in diameter, on echocardiography and the left shunt was patent.

At 12 years of age LV(left ventricular) ejection fraction(Simpson's rule) was 46%.Left shunt was patent but patient was hypoxic, and symptomatic. A right shunt was performed with significant improvement.

She did not show up for periodic examinations until 16 years of age, when she appeared again with dyspnea on exertion, increasing cyanosis, shortness of breath, and hemoptysis. She was deeply blue but two shunts were patent but inadequate in size. Recatheterization showed small left pulmonary artery with mutiple collaterals and a small patent shunt. The right pulmonary artery showed origin stensosis and a small patent right shunt.Aotric pO^2 was 48 mmHg and saturation was 86%. Bilateral pulmonary artery origin stenosis was again noted. The patient was not suitable for univentricular repair (Fontan operation). Therefore a right central shunt was performed. She did well postoperatively, with oxygen saturation 80 %.

At 19 years of age she reappeared deeply cyanotic with shortness of breath, headaches and fatigue. O^2 saturation was 65% (pulse oximetry). Left ventricular dysfunction (ejection fraction 40%) and heart failure (NTproBNP 270 pg/ml) were present.

At her last clinic visit at the age of 23 years, after not accepting to be considered for heart-lung transplantation, she was in poor clinical shape with severe hypoxia and left ventricular failure.

A CT angio was performed, to re-evaluate her pulmonary artery system and recommending a right Glenn shunt.

This study shows the strength of CT angiography in showing details of a complex anomaly of the pulmonary arteries.

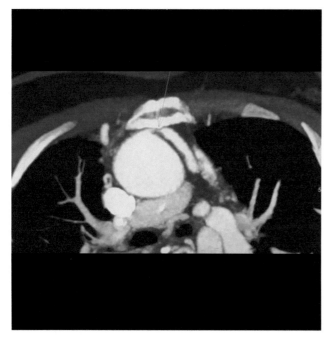

Figure 50: Note arrow pointing to the kinked origin of the central shunt from the aorta.

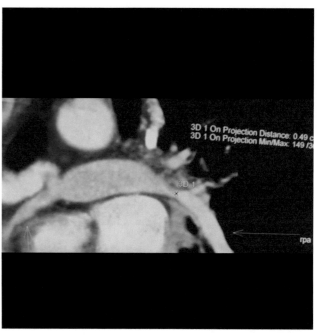

Figure 52: Nonconfluent RPA(right pulmonary artery) with stenosis (0.49 cm) distal to the shunt site.

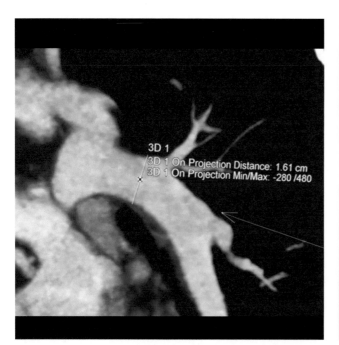

Figure 51: Note nonconfluent pulmonary artery, with a hypoplastic LPA and a left subclavian artery shunt. Alos see next figure.

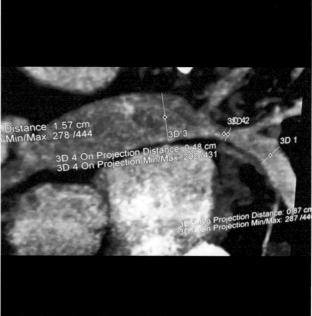

Figure 53: Figure 52:Detailed measurements of the nonconfluent RPA.

Case study: IBS #003

The patient is a 5-year-old boy referred by his pediatrician with a diagnosis of Kawasaki disease. Physical examination, EKG and echocardiography were within normal limits. RCA (right coronary artery) origin measured 0.17 mm and LCA (left coronary artery) origin measured 0.31 mm on echocardiogram. Because of patient's private physician's insistence a CT angio was performed to rule out any coronary artery lesion. This study shows normal coronary arteries.

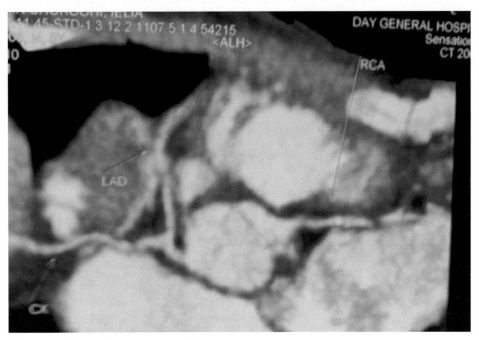

Figure 54: Normal coronary arteries.

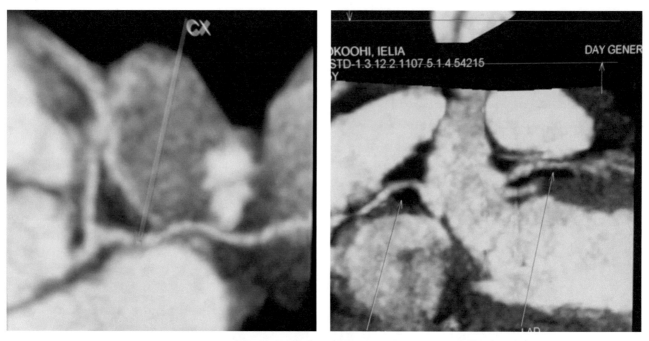

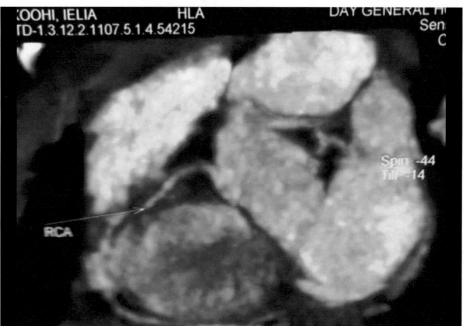

Figure 55: RCA (right coronary artery);CX (circumflex);LAD (left anterior descending coronary artery).

Case study:ARBZ #004

The patient was first seen at 3 years of age. A precordial systolic murmur was noted in infancy. Patient showed features of Silver dwarfism. EKG showed mild RVH(right ventricular hypertrophy). Echocardiography showed bicuspid aortic valve,with mild AS(aortic stenosis) (20 mmHg) and minimal AR (aortic regurgitation).On yearly follow-ups his aortic stenosis progressed gradually. At 12 yrs of age aortic valve stenosis peak gradient was 25 mmHg. At 13 years of age AS peak gradient was 33 mmHg. At 14 years of age aortic stenosis was 37-40 mmHg and EKG showed LVH (left ventricular hypertrophy) with increased posterior forces. At 15 years of age echocardiography showed thick bicuspid aortic valve with peak gradient 44 mmHg. Ascending aorta was dilated (2.72 cm in diameter). LVH was present IVSd (ventricular septum in diastole) thickness 1.2 cm. IVSs(ventricular septum in systole) thickness 1.7 cm, LVPWs(left ventricular posterior wall thickness in systole) was 1.7-1.9 cm. and LVPWd (left ventricular posterior wall thickness in diastole) thickness was1.31 cm.

A CT angio was performed prior to operation.

Eventually patient underwent aortic valvotomy at 15 1/2 years of age with peak systolic gradient of 44-47 mmHg.Postoperatively aortic valve peak gradient was 14-20 mmHg.

On his last exam he is 18 1/2 years of age. Obese with aortic valve peak gradient 20-22mmHg, and trivial AR. CT angio:

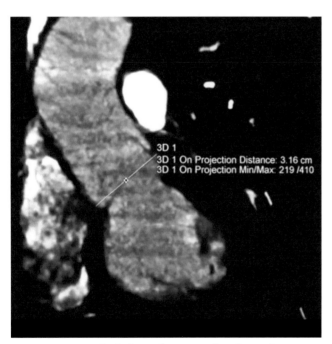 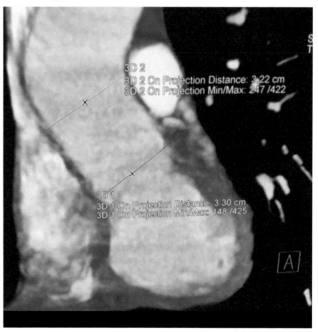

Figure 56: Note thick domed aortic valve above the measurement line.

Figure 57: Note LVH(left ventricular hypertrophy) and dilated ascending aorta

Case study: MC #005

Patient a 45-day-old boy was diagnosed to have tricupid atresia type IB,ie no transposition with pulmonary stenosis (PS).A left shunt was performed because of severe PS and cyanosis.The shunt clotted and it was reopened by the surgeon within the first 24 hours. At nine months of age the patient had acquired pulmonary atresia and atrial septum was aneurysmal. At 2 years of age left shunt was patent. LPA (left pulmonary artery) measured 0.98 and RPA(right pulmonary artery) meassured 0.77 mm in diameter. Patient had 2 SVCs (superior venae cavae).A right and left Glenn were performed and the left shunt was ligated at 26 mos of age.

CT angio was performed when the patient was 4 years old, in preparation for a tunnel with fenestrum (Fontan operation).

This study showed tricuspid atresia, VSD(ventricular septal defect), minuscule RV(right ventricle), an enlarged RA (right atrium) and a well developed LV(left ventricle.Acquired pulmonary artery atresia was noted. RSVC(right superior vena cava) drained into the RPA (right pulmonary artery), LSVC(left superior vena cava) drained into the proximal RPA. LPA (left pulmonary artery) was cut off at origin to a lenght of 1.3 cm. LPA diameter was 0.47 cm.

Retrospectively after the left shunt clotted and it was revised by the surgeon the proximal LPA also clotted thus the CT angio findings explain the cause of interrupted LPA. Although the case for tunnel anastomosis was defunct, on the insistence of parents and the surgeon's hope to reconstruct LPA, the patient underwent operation and a Dacron graft was interposed on the LPA and MPA(main pulmonary artery).However postoperatively gross CNS (central nervous system) damage was noted and the patient expired a month after operation with enterobacter sepsis and DIC (diffuse intravascular coagulation).

CT angio frames:

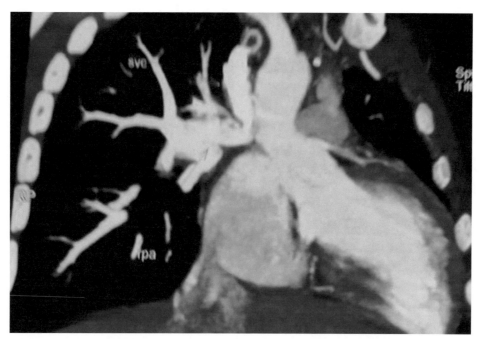

Figure 58: Note RSVC (right superior vena cava) on the right side of the aorta draining into the RPA (Rt Glenn).

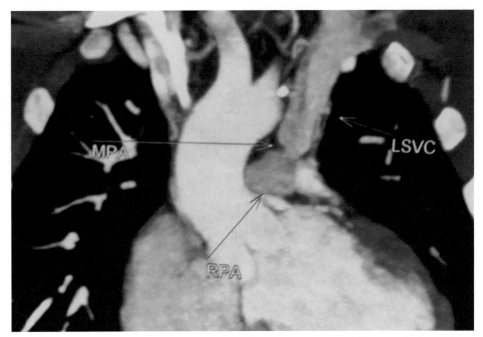

Figure 59: Note Left SVC draining into the proximal portion of the RPA (Bilateral Glenn shunts.)

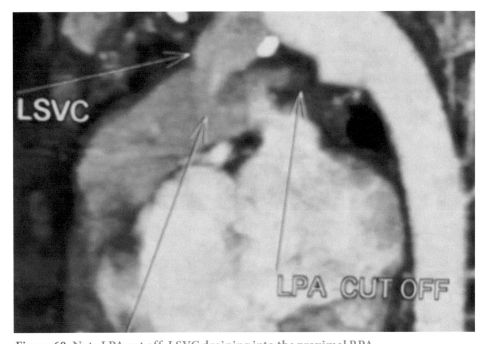

Figure 60: Note LPA cut off. LSVC draining into the proximal RPA.

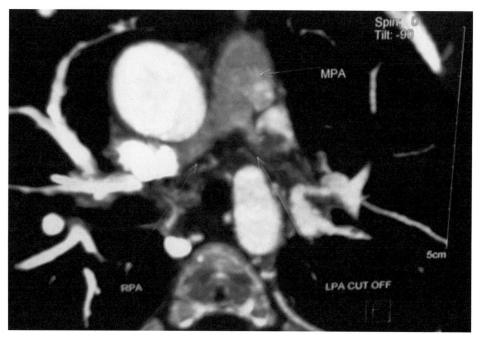

Figure 61: Note MPA at top middle, RPA,arrow on the left side of figure. LPA cut off
(right arrow) with 3 cm gap to the distal left inferior PA.

Case study :EAA# 006

The patient was first seen at 2 1/2 years of age with diagnosis of bicuspid aortic valve and aortic stenosis. He did not follow periodic exmaninations. On his last exam at 18 years of age his chief complaint was dyspnea during a football game. He had a grade 3/6 SEM(systolic ejection murmur) at LUSB (left upper sternal border) with EKG showing LVH (left ventricular hypertrophy) by voltage criteria. Echocardiography showed bicuspid aortic valve with LVH and PG (peak gradient) of 75 mmHg. A CT-angio was performed :

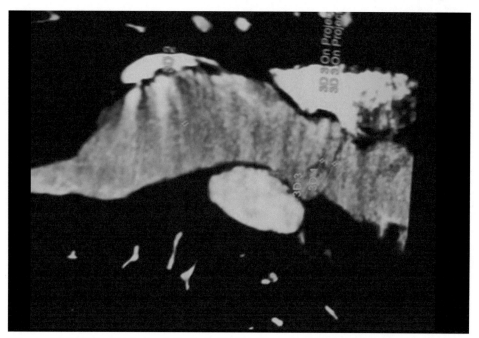

Figure 62: Thick aortic valve. Aortic orifice 2.52 cm. Dilated ascending aorta
3.64 cm.

Case study:HF#007

This 16-yr-old male with discrete coarctation of the aorta was operated after the first visit. He did fine. He was recatheterized at 27 yrs of age. This study showed dilated ascending aorta and aortic arch, with mismatch in size at the isthmus. Ascending aortic pressure was 135/95 mmHg and descending aortic pressure was 140/95 mmHg. At 29 years of age he had 25 mmHg peak gradient across the aortic isthmus by Doppler study.Recatheterized again when 30 years of age. At this time the patient was obese and hypertensive. Maximum 30 mmHg peak gradient was detected on catheterization, at the aortic isthmus at the junction of the aortic arch, left subclavian and descending aorta. At 32 years of age again patient was obese, hypertensive and had 35 mmHg peak gradient by Doppler study at the aortic isthmus. The site of stenosis was neither amenable to stent procedure nor the job of a cardiac surgeon.A vascular surgeon for approaching this problem was the best option.

CT angio showed the site of obstruction with the proximal isthmus of the aorta dilated.

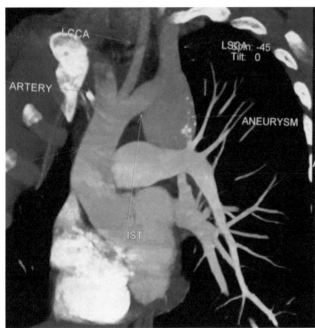

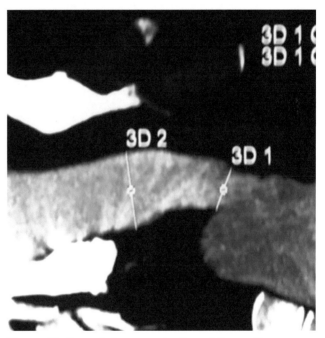

Figure 63: LAO view of the aortic arch.Note left subclavian artery, left common carotid artery, right innominate artery and small bright origin of the internal mammary artery arising from the aortic arch from left to right. Note the site of recoarctation (arrow). The aortic isthmus is aneurysmal.

Figure 64: Curved planar projection of the aortic pathology. 3D1 1.49 cm in diameter, site of recoarctation. 3D2 aortic arch just before coarctation measures 2.66 cm. Note aneurysmally dilated aortic isthmus below recoarctation.

The patient was recommended to seek help abroad, preferably at a center with expertise in complex vascular surgery. However at 34 years of age he went to Germany where the isthmus was stented,with a peak gradient of 14 mmHg by Doppler post-procedure. Following the procedure he had dissecting aortic aneurysm. Therefore he was operated and another stent was implanted in the aorta distal to the coarctation site and a tube graft was inserted between left subclavian artery and the aortic isthmus distal to the stent, because the ostium of the left subclavian artery was occluded by the first stent.

At this time 25 mmHg peak gradient existed in the descending aorta.

To recheck the anatomy **CT angio** was repeated.

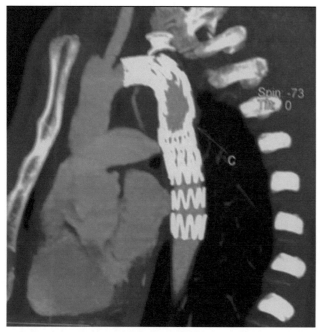

Figure 65: Sagittal view of the stented recoarcation and the dissected descending aortic aneurysm. Left subclavian artery obliterated and the graft nonfunctional.

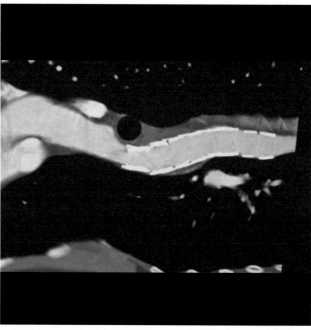

Figure 66: Curved planar view of the stented isthmus and descending aorta, with obliteration of the left subclavian artery.

The recoarctation stent distal to the left carotid artery was patent. The stent occluded the ostium of the left subclavian artery.The stent in the descending aorta distal to the coarctation site was patent.The left subclavian artery graft to the descending aorta graft was clotted.

Because the patient was clinically asymptomatic and left carotid flow was normal, further stenting the orifice of the left carotid,recommended in Germany, was cancelled.

Case study:MZEM #008

Patient was first seen at 11 months of age with tetralogy of Fallot and blue spells. Patient has one normal sister and he has followed 5 miscarriages. Echocardiographically RVOT (right ventricular outfllow tract) was severely stenotic. MPA (main pulmonary artery) was 0.8 cm in diameter. LPA (left pulmonary artery) and RPA(right pulmonary artery) were 0.5 and 0.4 cm in diameter respectively. A left shunt was performed. Patient showed up at 2 years of age at which time he had elfine features (infantile hypercalcemia), and because he was hypoxic again a catheterization was performed which showed small pulmonary arterial system. Subsequently a right shunt was performed. LPA measured 0.8 and RPA was 1.01 cm in diameter.At 3 years of age he was recatheterized, however total correction was deferred because of small PA (pulmopnary artery) size.

At 6 years of age he was recatheterized and total correction was recommended, however the patient went elsewhere for surgical repair and did not show up until he was 8 years of age.At this time he was in heart failure. His heart was grossly enlarged. Echocardiography showed moderate TR(tricuspid regurgitation) with peak gradient of 35 mmHg, RA(right atrial) volume 73ml/m^2; severe pulmonary regurgitation and grossly dilated RVOT(right ventricular outflow tract).The patient was in severe heart failure with NTproBNP 2062pg/ml. A CT angio was performed:

CT angio: showed 1-severe LPA bifurcation stenosis 2- a right scimitar syndrome,ie right lower lobe pulmonary vein draining into the IVC(inferior vena cava). 3-a collateral at T12 to the RLL. 4- Grossly dilated right ventricle.

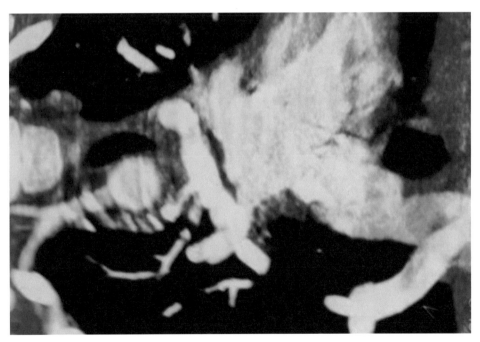

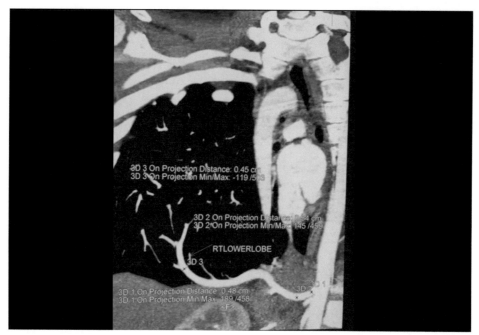

Figure 67: Collateral artery at T12 to the right lower lobe.

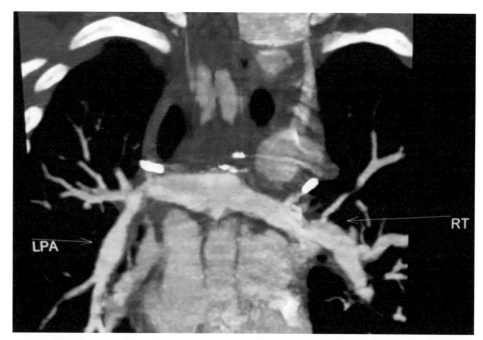

Figure 68: Posterior view,showing severe LPA bifurcation stenosis.RPA 1.05 cm, LPA 1.02 cm, and LPA bifurcation 0.46 cm in diameter respectively.

Progress Report:

Total correction of defects were recommended. The patient could not afford private hospital charges and he was eventually operated elsewhere at 9 years of age.**CT angio post-second repair showed:**

1-LPA bifurcation stenosis was not be repaired. 2- RVOT (right ventricular outflow tract) was repaired. 3- A #21 Medtronic porcine valve was implanted for pulmonic valve .4-Scimitar, and the collateral at T12 were not tackled.

At another hospital it was claimed that the scimitar vessel was occluded. The LPA was not stented because there was no stenosis [cath showed RV pressure of 80 mmHg,and PA pressure of 45 mmHg!!] and the collateral to the right lower lobe was not occluded.

At last visit at 11 years of age the patient was in severe heart failure with systemic pressure in RV(right ventricle).The porcine valve was degenerated and severely stenotic.LPA(left pulmonary artery) bifurcation stenosis persisted. RVOT was grossly dilated. There was severe cardiomegaly and severe heart failure attested to by an NTproBNP level of 1669 pg/ml.The patient was terminal and was on symptomatic treatment.

Case study:AMN #009

Patient was first seen at the age of 18 mos. Congenital heart disease wasd diagnosed at 9 months of age. The patient was in heart failure.EKG showed first degree AV block, QRS axis 100 degrees. QS in V1-V5,all posterior forces. The heart was enlarged and pulmonary vascular markings were increased on chest X-ray. On echocardiography LTGV(L transposition of the great vessels) was noted with large VSD(ventricular septal defect), and ASD (atrial septal defect) .The VSD showed no gradient and PR (pulmonary regurgitation) was 25 mmHg. Cardiac catheterization confirmed the above findings.Massive TR(tricuspid regurgitation) on the left side was noted. PA (pulmonary artery) pressure was 85/50(mean60) mmHg.After medical therapy PA banding was recommended at high risk. PA banding was performed with gradient of 56 mmHg. Severe TR persisted.At 2 year of age PAB (pulmonary artery band) peak gradient was 63 mmHg by Doppler. He underwent VSD and ASD closure,PA was debanded. A small residual VSD was present. TR was significantly improved. TR peak gradient was 45 mmHg and mild subpulmonary stenosis peak gradient, 34 mmHg developed at 3 years of age.At 3 years of age he showed severe sub-pulmonary stenosis with 67 mmHg peak gradient by Doppler .

CT angio: situs solitus, LTGV,

This study shows L-TGV, ie aortic valve is anterior, superior to the left and pulmonic valve is inferior posterior and to the right of the aortic root (Frames 1 and 2).There is severe subpulmonary stenosis with site of PAB shown on lateral frame.The ventricle which feeds pulmonary artery is smooth inside (ie left ventricle feeds the pulmonary artery).SVC(superior vena cava) drains into right sided RA(right atrium), which is connected to the anatomic LV(left ventricle) (smooth inside), feeding the pulmonary artery. RV(right ventricle) is connected to the aorta to the left and LV(left ventricle) is connected to the PA(pulmonary artery).

This late onset subpulmonary stenosis is called the Gasul phenomenon which is sometimes noted in patients with VSD.

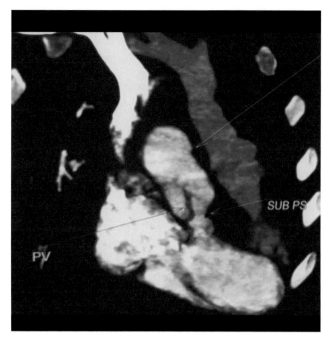

Figure 69: Note aortic valve (anterior) superior to the left, and pulmonic valve(posterior) inferior to the right,originating from a smooth-walled LV, thus LTGV .

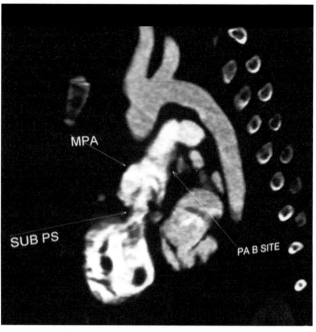

Figure 71: This frame shows thick pulmonic valve plus severe subpulmonary stenosis, and site of repair of the previous PA band.

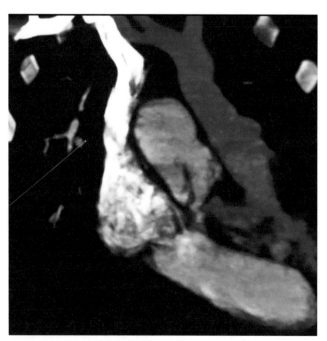

Figure 70: From left to right: SVC drains into the RA, which is connected to a smooth walled LV giving rise to the PA, ie LTGV. To the right a heavily trabeculated RV is connected to the aorta to the left, ie LTGV.

The patient underwent tube graft #22 conduit with biologic Edward valve for relief of subpulmonary stenosis at 4 1/2 years of age.

At 6 year of age, the biologic valve shows mild PR(pulmonary regurgitation),and has 12 mmHg peak gradient in systole.

At 7 years of age the Edward valve is degenerating. Also there is moderate right sided MR (mitral regurgitation) and mild left-sided TR (tricuspid regurgitation) .

At 8 yrs of age the valve is degenerated, PG (peak gradient) 18 mmHg,PR +++,MR+++,TR+++, and we are trying to buy time for polyvalvar surgery!!

Case study:KK#252

The patient is a 5-year-old girl followed since 3 years of age,with diagnosis of restrictive cardiomyopathy, heart failure and failure to thrive. A prominent S4 on auscultation,was due to gross right atrial enlargement. EKG showed giant P waves with biatrial hypertrophy, increased posterior forces and gross ST elevation in V4R, V1 and V2. Echocardiography showed moderate systolic dysfunction, and gross diastolic dysfunction. The pericardium looked thick and shiny. To rule out constrictive pericarditis a CT angio was performed. This study showed thin pericardium and no evidence to support constrictive pericarditis. Final diagnosis: restrictive cardiomyopathy.

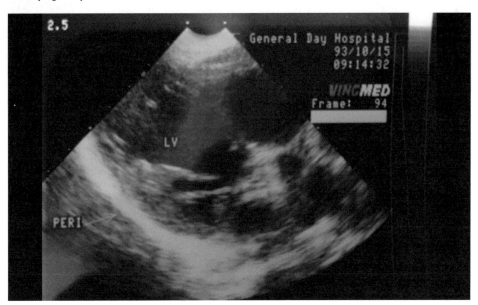

Figure 72: Echocardiogram, long axis view showing thick, shiny pericardium

CT angio frame shows enlarged RA.No evidence to support constrictive pericarditis. Pericardium is thin.

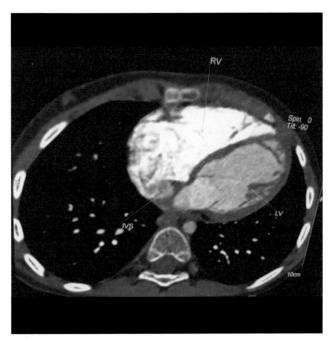

Figure 73: CT angio frame showing large RA(right atrium), pericardium thin and normal.

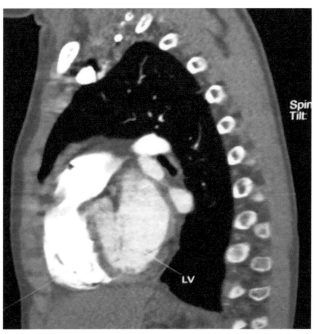

Figure 74: Note thin pericardium anteriorly and posteriorly.

Case study:MY#219

Patient a 12.5-year-old female opertated first at 37 days of age for severe valvar aortic stenosis.A membranous VSD closed spontaneously. The aortic valve was bicuspid. Again she was operated for coarctation of the aorta at 18 months of age.Postoperatively there was mild aortic stenosis with peak gradient by Doppler of 25 mmHg. At 12.5 years of age she had 35 mmHg peak gradient in the descending aorta. However clinically the femoral pulses were normal and blood pressure was 110/65 mmHg in the right arm in supine position. CT angio was performed to rule out recoarctation.

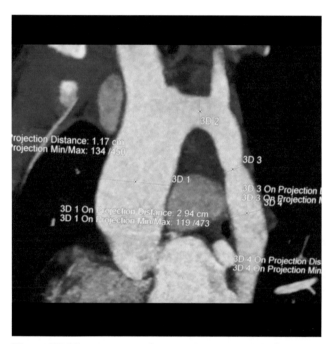

Figure 75: Note segmental narrowing at aortic isthmus, 0.80 cm in diameter,however there is no obstruction.

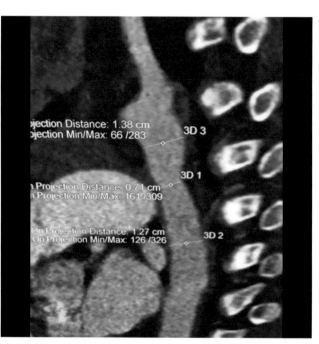

Figure 76: Curved planar presentation of the ascending aorta,isthmus and descending aorta. Note segmental narrowing of the isthmus 0.71 cmin diameter.

This study ruled out recoarctation.

The problem of false echo-derived gradient from the aortic isthmus must be recognized. A diagnosis of recoarctation must not be made only by an echo-derived pressure gradient. If the clinical examination shows nomal blood pressure in the right arm, and if the femoral pulses are normal, the Doppler derived gradient should be ignored. A CT angio will confirm the clinical diagnosis of pseudocoarctation by Doppler, and the need for catheterization is obviated.

Baumgartner et al's report on the effect of stenosis geometry on the Doppler-catheter gradient relation in vitro is most instructive.See reference section under coarctation of the aorta.

Another example of this phenomenon is shown below|:

Case study: ML #159

The patient is a 16-year -old boy followed since 3 years of age. He had coarctation of the aorta,which was corrected by end-to-end anastomosis shortly after the first visit. Preoperative echo-derived peak gradient was 70 mmHg. At 13 years of age he showed a peak gradient of 40 mmHg by Doppler, however his blood pressure was within normal limits and femoral pulses were normal in amplitude.

The following CT angio frame shows that the basis for Doppler-derived pressure gradient was incongruity of the diameter of the various segments of the aortic arch and isthmus.

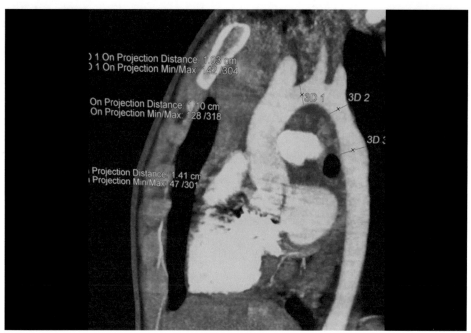

Figure 77: Aortic arch 1.03, proximal isthmus 1.10,distal isthmus 1.41 cm in diameter respectively. No recoarctation.

Case study:FM#031

Patient was first seen at 3 days of age with, a spectrum of tricuspid atresia type IA,ie hypoplastic RV(right ventricle), a small TV (tricuspid valve),a restrictive VSD (ventricular septal defect),pulmonary atresia, and a small PDA(patent ductus arteriosus). At 6 months of age she underwent a right BT(Blalock-Taussig) shunt. Recatheterization at 5 years of age showed suprasystemic RV pressure, right-to-left shunt via an ASD(atrial septal defect).Pulmonary arterial system was found unsuitable for Fontan operation. At 6 years of age she had a right central shunt for severe hypoxia.

At 14.5 years of age she was deeply cyanotic. She was catheterized and again found unsuitable for Fontan operation.A third shunt was performed on the left side.Pulse oximetry showed improved oxygenation, 84% O2 saturation.

A CT angio was performed at 19 years of age. This study showed pulmonary atresia with confluent pulmonary arterial system. Hypoplasia of the main, right and left pulmonary arteries was noted, however the peripheral branches were of almost normal size. The right BT shunt was patent and last shunt on the left pulmonary artery was patent. The left central shunt was clotted. There was a substernal aortic pseudoaneurysm at the level of the 2nd sternal suture. Plan was to ligate the aortic pseudoaneurysm, ligate the right pulmonary artery, leaving the shunt alone and connecting IVC(inferior vena cava) to the LPA(left pulmonary artery) using a tunnel with fenestrum to the RA(right atrium) and enlarge the ASD. Father declined any further procedures and the patient was lost to follow-up.

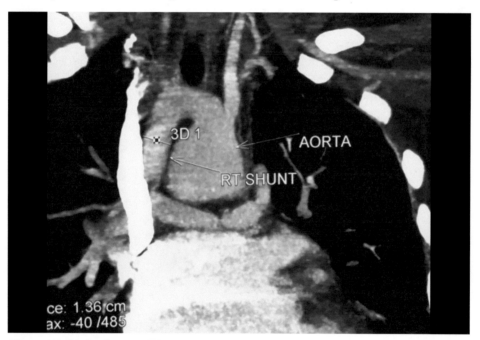

Figure 78: Right shunt on RPA

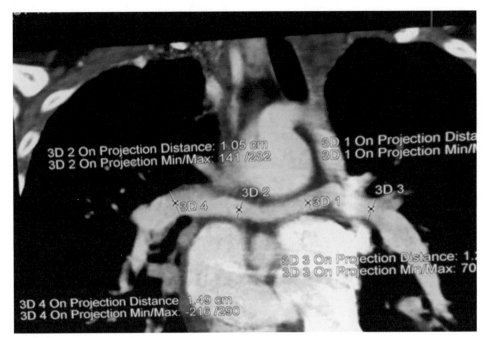

Figure 79: RPA,proximal 1.05,distal 1.49 cm respectively;LPA proximal 1.00, distal1.27 cm respectively.

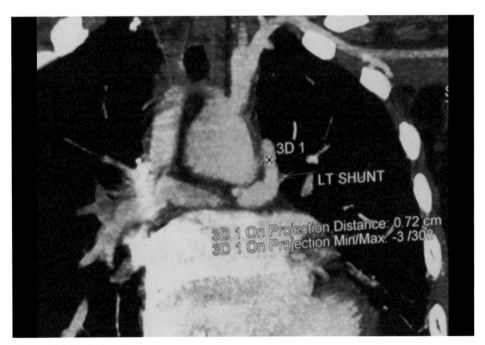

Figure 80: Left shunt.

Case study:KM#011

Patient is a 2-month-old full-term boy who was referred for cyanosis and rapid breathing.He was diagnosed to have d-TGV(d-transposition of the great vessels), intact ventricular septum, a stretchted PFO (patent foramen ovale) and a small PDA(patent ductus arteriosus).Emergency BH (Blalock-Hanlon) procedure was performed. At 8 months of age he had 32 mmHg flow gradient in the PA (pulmonary artery), the BH was quite large, and he had mild TR (tricuspid regurgitation). At 14 months of age he had severe TR with enlarged heart and CHF(congestive heart failure). NTproBNP was 747 pg/ml.A PA(pulmonary artery) banding was performed at 14 months of age. The following CT angio was performed prior to arterial switch.

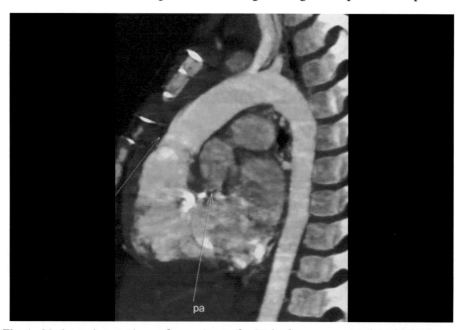

Figure 81: Aorta is anterior and superior to the PA(pulmonary artery),ie dTGV in situs solitus.PA band is seen as a stricture above the pulmonic valve.

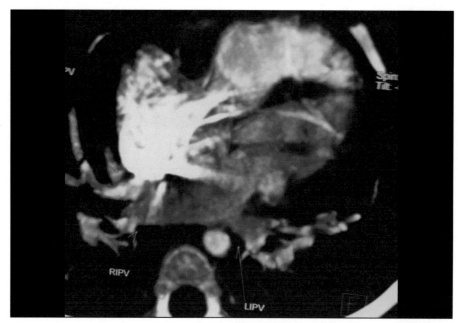

Figure 82: RV (right ventricle)is anterior and LV (left ventricle) postrerior. The ventricular septum is intact. All 4 pulmonary veins drain normally into the LA(left atrium).

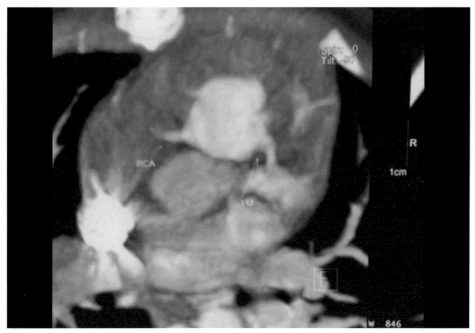

Figure 83: Aorta in the middle with normal main coronary arteries on cross section. LA(left atrium) and PVs(pulmonary veins) are seen posteriorly.

Arterial switch, closure of BH defect and PA-debanding were performed at 20 months of age.Post-operatively the patient expired due to DIC (diffuse intravascular coagulation).

Case study: AJ #012

Seven-year-old boy with homocystinuria, severe kyphoscoliosis, biventricular CMP(cardiomyopathy), and aneurysmal ascending aorta and mild AR(aortic regurgitation).By age 12 years he had massive AR. A CT angio confirmed the above findings. He underwent AVR (aortic valve replacement) #25 Carbomedics, ascending aorta replacement and coronary re-implantation.Presently he is 16 years of age.He has CMP and is up for spine surgery.

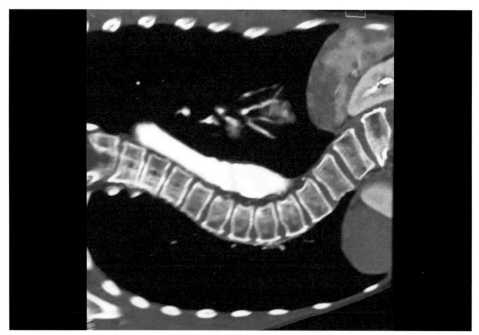

Figure 84: Severe kyphoscoliosis.

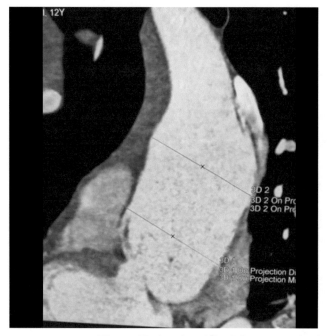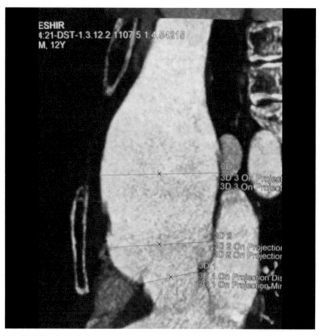

Figure 85: Aortic orifice 2.84 cm, aortic sinus of Valsalva 5.31 cm, and ascending aorta aneurysm 5.84 cm in diameter.

Case study: MA: #018:

Adult patients with congenital heart disease, may need reoperation . One exampler is that of tetralogy of Fallot corrected in infancy or childhood. Over the years these patients may develop RV(right ventricular) failure secondary to pulmonary regurgitation and/or RVOT(right ventricular outflow tract) patch aneurysm. Especially those patients who have had transannular patch are be prone to RV dysfunction. While studying these patients for repair of the RVOT patch aneurym and pulmonary valve replacement, their coronary arteries should be looked at to rule out CAD(coronary artery disease), which could confront the patient with serious problems during or after reoperation for CHD(congenital heart disease).

This case is a 32-yr-old man, married with 2 children who needs such an operation. His coronaries were also studied by CT angiography, together with his CHD, prior to embarking on pulmonic valve replacement and RVOT repair for severe PR(pulmonary regurgitation) and RVOT aneuysm. The astute radiologist may detect problems, never diagnosed before. In this particular patient, left hydronephrosis, and degeneration of several spinal discs were diagnosed.

The following frames show normal coronary arteries.

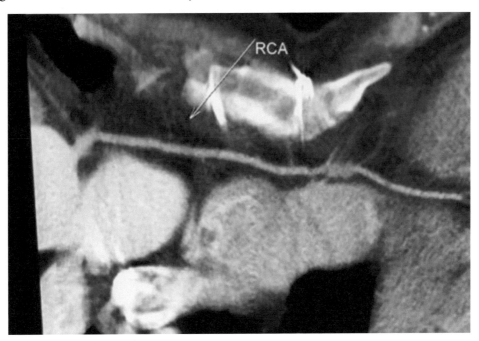

Figure 86: Note normal RCA.

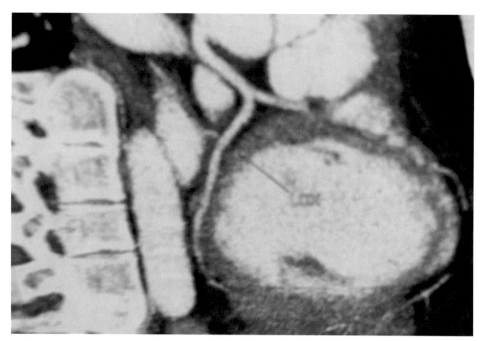

Figure 87: Note normal LCX, and degenerated intervertebral discs.

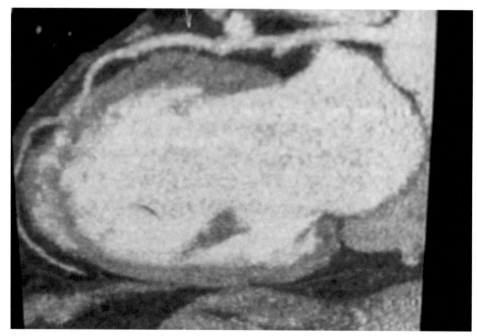

Figure 88: Note normal LAD coronary artery.

Case study: MN #253

The patient is a 47-year-old female followed since 30 years of age. Congenital heart disease was diagnosed at 29 years of age.She is married and has a normal son. She had C-TGV(corrected transposition of the great vessels), a VSD (ventricular septal defect) which closed spontaneously.At 40 years of age she developed TR(tricuspid regurgitation).When 43 years old, she had hysterectomy.

Over the years, she developed systemic hypertension.Not obese, not diabetic, she complained of chest pain, and dyspnea on exertion. EKG showed NSR (normal sinus rhythm),at a rate of 90/min.QRS axis was at -60 degrees.PR-interval was prolonged 180 ms,QS complexes noted in V4R, and V1 consistent with C-TGV.Increased posterior forces, negative T-waves in lead I and aVL. Patient is hypertensive.Left-sided RV EF(right ventricular ejection fraction) 43%(Simpson), with moderatge left-sided TR. An exercise test showed suboptimal results with PVCs,BP 170/90, at 10.4 METs and ST-segment elevation.

A CT angio was performed to rule out major coronary artery disease. This study showed that major coronary arteries were within normal limits, and no obstructions were noted. Therefore the patient's complaints and clinical findings were due to myocardial microcirculatory insufficiency.

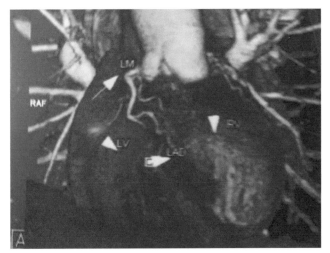

Figure 89: Note RCA and LM and LAD, reverse of normal. Aorta originates from the right ventricle.

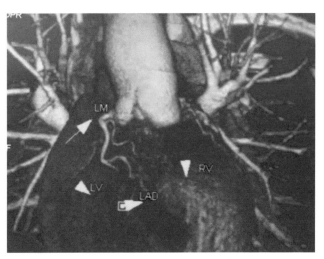

Figure 90: Note LTGV, aorta originating from RV. Coronaries are in reverse fashion of normal.

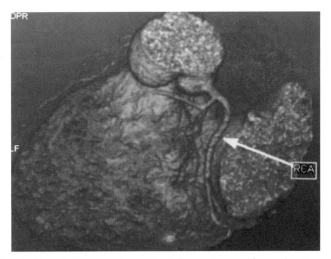

Figure 91: Note RCA originating above the left aortic cusp from the sinus of Valsalva and LM originating above the right aortic valve cusp.

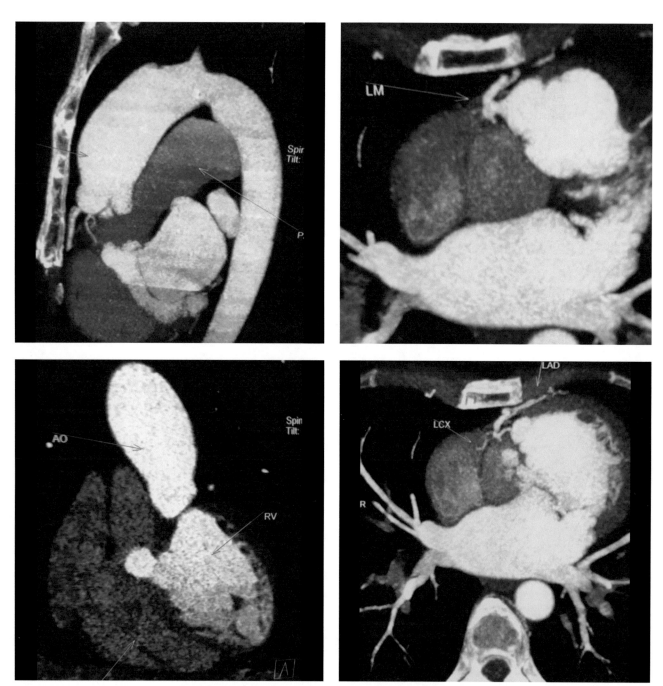

Figure 92: Left-sided RV,heavily trabeculated with a conus giving rise to the aorta (LTGV).Note a septal aneurysm closing a membranous VSD.

Figure 93: Note LM (left main) coronary artery (top frame) giving rise to LAD and LCX (bttom frame) arising from above the right aortic cusp from the sinus of Valsalva.

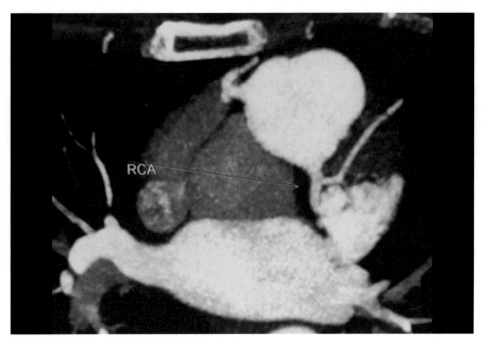

Figure 94: Note RCA arising above the left aortic cusp.

Case study: AT#012

This patient presented at 5 days of age with respiratory distress and heart failure.He showed isolated levocardia on chest-X Ray. Once a diagnosis of **isolated levocardia, or Ivemark's syndrome** is made one knows for sure that one is dealing with complex heart disease. This patient had DORV (double outlet right ventricle) with d-TGV(transposition of the great vessels), pulmonary valvar and subvalvar stenosis, large sinus venosus ASD (atrial septal defect), mitral atresia and a hypoplastic LV(left ventricle), on echocardiographic examination.

Note situs ambiguus on figure 2, which belongs to this patient.

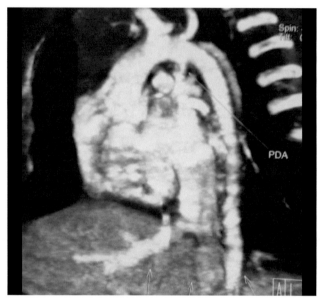

Figure 95: Note dTGV, anterior aorta arising from the large right ventricle. A PDA(patent ductus arteriosus) feeds the PA (pulmonary artery) which is posterior in position.

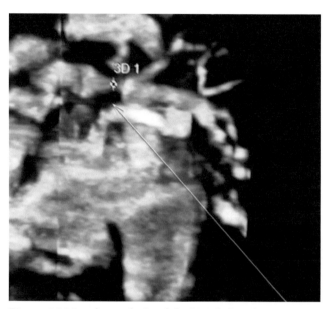

Figure 96: Note hypoplasia of the LPA(left pulmonary artery) with origin stenosis (arrow).

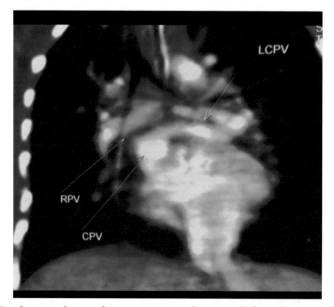

Figure 97: Total anomalous pulmonary venous drainage:left and right common pulmonary veins join to form common pulmonary vein draining into thelower part of the SVC (superior vena cava).

Case study: HN # 020

This 26-day-old girl presented with severe heart failure, a massively enlarged heart and gross RVH (right ventricular hypertrophy) on the EKG. Situs solitus, and almost a common atrium were diagnosed with TAPVD into the high right atrium. A CT angio was performed, which confirmed the dignosis.

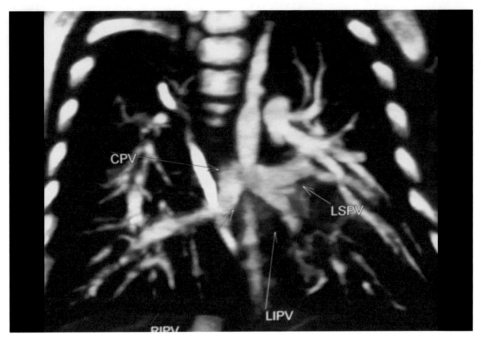

Figure 98: Note right and left inferior pulmonary veins, joining the common pulmonary vein, draining into the low SVC (superior vena cava).

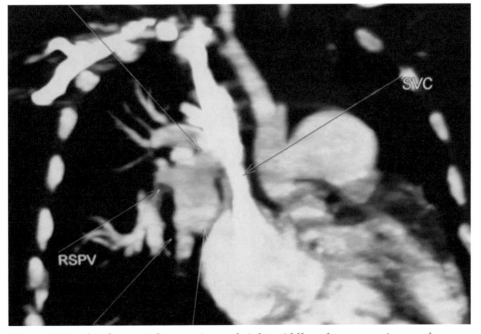

Figure 99: In this frame right superior and right middle pulmonary veins are shown joining the common pulmonary vein, draining into the low SVC.

Case study: BB #023

The patient was first seen at the age of 20 months.She was diagnosed to have CHD(congenital heart disease) and had undergone a left Goretex shunt.She was blue and had dextrocardia on chest X-ray, but she had situs solitus on EKG and chest X-ray. Echocardiography showed situs solitus, dextrocardia,LV(left ventricle) was right sided and RV(right ventricle) was left sided. There was pulmonary atresia and aorta originated from the anatomic RV(right ventricle) on the left side. The shunt was clotted and there was a PDA (patent ductus arteriosus). A right shunt was performed at 21 months of age,with good result. At age 4 1/2 years, she had a CT angio prior to total correction. This study showed situs solitus, dextro-,/mesocardia, RA(right atrium) to the right, LA(left atrium) to the left. LV (left ventricle) was to the right, RV(right ventricle) was to the left. There was pulmonary atresia. Aorta originated from the left-sided RV(right ventricle) and MPA(main pulmonary artery) was atretic. Right and left pulmonary arteries were confluent. Left shunt was clotted and right shunt was patent.

She had Rastelli operation in Germany.The VSD was enlarged with pericardial patch and aorta was connected to right sided LV(left ventricle). A Contegra, 20 mm bovine xenograft was used to connect the left sided RV(right ventricle) to the PA(pulmonary artery). Postoperatively she had subdural hematoma,from which she recovered without CNS sequelae, however she had severe, relentless CHF (congestive heart failure) withNTpro-BNP 4689 pg/ml.The LV-RA shunt peak gradient was 54 by Doppler. Right atrial volume index was 45 ml/m². She had a false route, between LV(left ventricle) and RA(right atrium) causing massive shunt, right atrial enlargement and severe heart failure. Surgical closure of the iatrogenic LV-RA shunt was recommended. The patient disappeared and never showed up again.

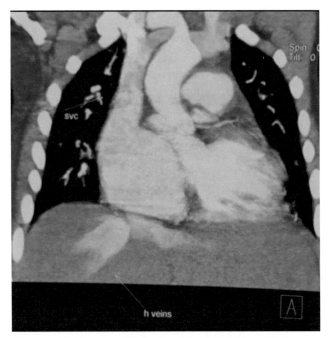

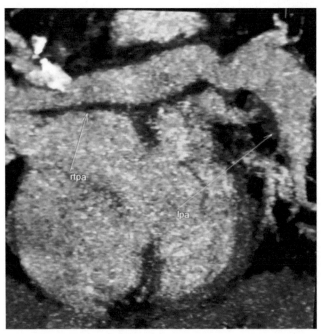

Figure 100: Liver, and hepatic veins and IVC on the right. This means situs solitus with dextro/mesocardia.So RA is right-sided. Aorta originated from left-sided RV with a conus,therefore we have l-loop,with TGV.

Figure 101: Note pulmonary atresia,with confluent right and left pulmonary arteries.

Case study: MNF #026

Patient is a 3 1/2- year-old-boy who was catheterized and diagnosed to have agenesis of the RPA (right pulmonary artery) and tetralogy of Fallot with absent pulmonic valve, right aortic arch and microscopic pulmonary AV(arteriovenous) fistulas.He had total correction in October 1989, at Deborrah Heart Center, New Jersey, USA at the age of 6 years. A 19 mm porcine xenograft was used for the RVOT (right ventricular outflow tract), and VSD(ventricular septal defect) was closed. He was erratic in follow-up appointments and taking medications.He was catheterized by the author, at the age of 23 years and he was found to have a dilated aneurysmal LPA (left pulmonary artery) and a degenerated xenograft. His RV (right ventricular) pressure was 55-60 /10 mmHg. PA (pulmonary artery) pressure was 35/25 (mean 30) mmHg. His blood gas study in room air showed PaO2 of 58 mmHg and O2 saturation was 90 percent. Cyanosis and low PaO2 are due to R-L shunting in the left lung, due to Va/Q abnormality,most probably caused by microscopic pulmonary arteriovenous fistulas. LPA was aneurysmal. His RV was dysfunctional as shown by high RVEDP(right ventricular end-diastolic pressure).He had erratic follow-up. A CT angio was performed at age 25 years because of hemoptysis.At age 27 He had degenerated xenograft with peak systolic gradient of 30 mmHg by Doppler and moderate pulmonary xenograft regurgitation. He was in heart failure (NTproNP was 483 pg/ml).At 28 years of age his valve was grossly degenerated with peak systolic gradient over 40 mmHg peak,moderate to severe PR (pulmonary regurgitation), and mild to moderate TR (tricuspid regurgitation) with peak gradient of 67 mmHg by Doppler. He underwent reoperation at another hospital for changing the pulmonic valve,where he expired shortly after operation.

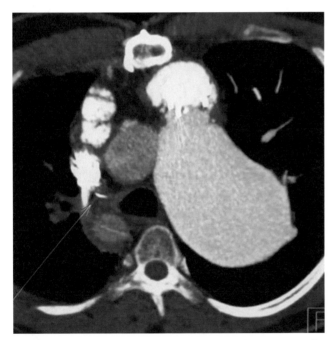

Figure 102: Note xenograft strut on top and aneurysmally dilated LPA (left pulmonary artery). Arrow at left bottom points to absent RPA(right pulmonary artery).

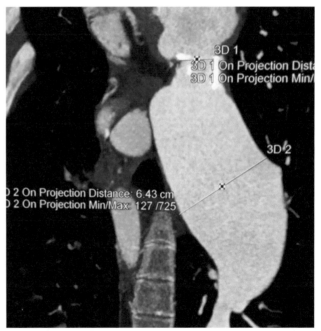

Figure 103: Curved planar view of the LPA(left pulmonary artery), aneurysmally dilated (6.84 cm in diameter) and segments of the descendingaorta to the right of the spine.

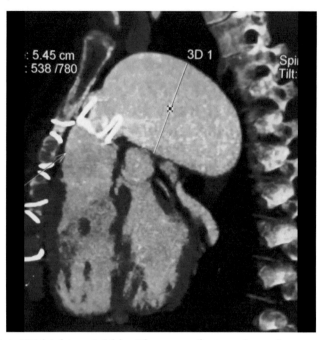

Figure 104: Note RV (right ventricle) with xenograft strut above the conus and aneurysmal LPA (left pulmonary artery)(5.45 cm in diameter).

Case study:AR # 027

Patient is an 18-year-old female followed since 2 days of age. A left atrial tumor was diagnosed by fetal echocardiography.The study was done because of arrhythmia of the fetal heart by the obstetrician.The patient is an obese girl with tuberous sclerosis, and mental-motor retardation. She is hypothyroid as well. At 8 months of age, cardiac examination showed multiple cardiac tumors. One in the RA(right atrium), one in the LA(left atrium), 3 in the LV(left ventricle), 2 in the RV (right ventricle) and RVOT(right ventricular outflow tract). Over the years several tumors gradually regressed in size. At 13 years of age a CT angio was performed.One apicolateral intracavitary tumor (1.36x0.91 cm) and one intramural apicolateral tumor (probably lipoma) were detected.The other tumors had been resorbed.

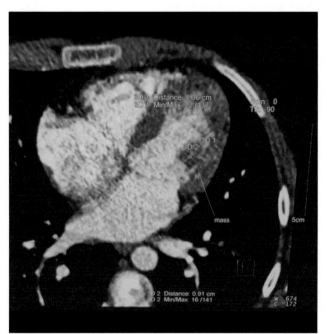
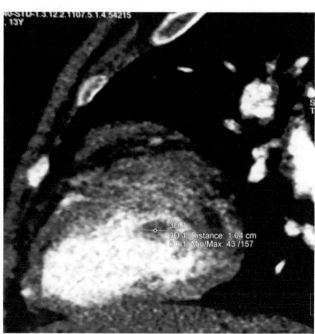

Figure 105: Note LV (left ventricular) intramural and and intracavitary masses.

Case study:AA # 029

The patient was first seen at the age of 31 years. He has situs inversus with meso-, or levocardia (Ivemark syndrome). At the age of 15 years he had a shunt done in England. Patient is erratic in follow-up visits. He was cyanotic and had clubbing of the finger-, and toe-nails. EKG showed situs inversus, left QRS axis at -80 degrees, and all posterior forces. Cardiac catheterization revealed situs inversus and isolated meso-, or levocardia, ie Ivemark syndrome with azygos continuation of IVC (inferior vena cava). Systemic veins entered the left-sided RA(right atrium) .An ASD (atrial septal defect) was present as well as partial anomalous pulmonary venous return. He had severe valvar, and subvalvar PS (pulmonary stenosis). Left shunt was patent and there were no collaterals feeding the lungs. RA(right atrium) was connected to the RV (right ventricle) on the left side and LA (left atrium) was connected to the LV(left ventricle) on the right side. A VSD (ventricular septal defect) in cushion position was present. Pulmonary artery originated from the left sided RV(right ventricle), and aorta (anterior to the right) originated from the LV(left ventricle) on the right side.

He had total correction of PAPVD(partial anomalous venous drainage),closure of the VSD(ventricular septal defect and relief of the pulmonary valvar and subpulmonary stenosis. However postoperatively he developed AF(atrial fibrillation).

On follow-up exams he did well, however he had multiple functional complaints especially chest pain. His AF was controlled for rate, however it never converted to sinus rhythm. Because echocardiography was physically impossible since after operation, a CT angio was performed at 33 years of age, to make sure of the anatomic correction, and the status of the coronary arteries.

The coronaries were within normal limits. Both LAD (on the left) and RCA(on the right) originated anteriorly from the aortic sinus of Valsalva.

The power of CT angio in delineating complex anomalies is shown below. Not only confirming the catheterization diagnosis, it added a very rare and fascinating anomaly in this case of Ivemark syndrome.

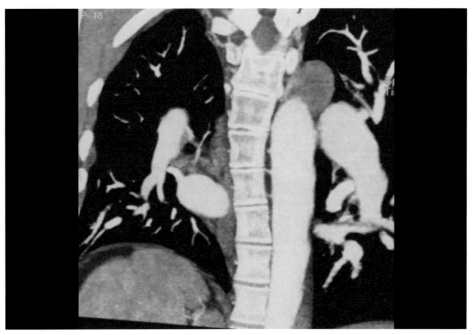

Figure 106: Azygos continuation of IVC (inferior vena cava), on the left side,ie situs inversus.

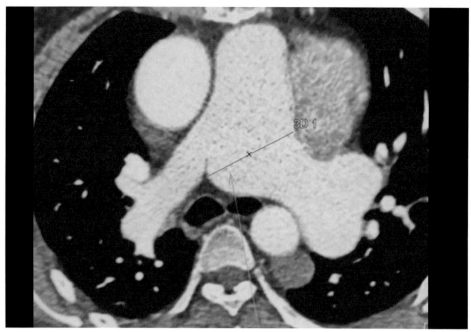

Figure 107: Note aneurysmally dilated LPA(left pulmonary artery). MPA(main pulmonary arter) 4.3 cm, RPA(right pulmonary artery) origin 2.02 cm, LPA origin 5.01 cm,LPA trunk 3.04 cm RVOT below the valve 2.12 cm.

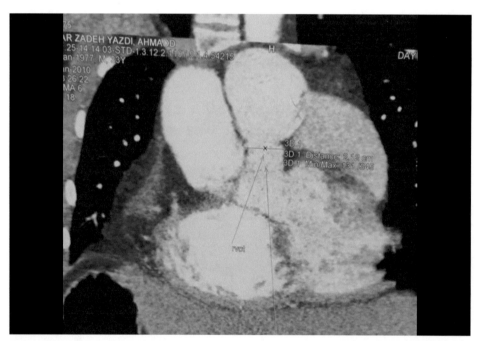

Figure 108: RV on the right giving rise to the PA. LV on the left giving rise to the Ao. So we have ILD ie situs inversus, L-loop of the ventricles and d-loop of the great vessels.

However this study sheds more light on the diagnosis. The following figure shows that both ventricles have conus. A very rare occurrence. See epilogue for the first case of subtruncal conus.

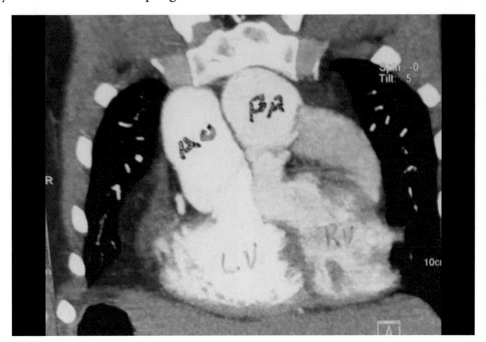

Figure 109: Note a conus underneath the thick pulmonic valve, and a smaller conus under the aortic valve on the right.

(See Epilogue.Truncus arteriosus with subtruncal conal growth.)

Case study:MAS # 041

Patient is a 28-year-old male who has been followed since 10 years of age with tetralogy of Fallot and pulmonary atresia. He had a right shunt as an infant and had subsequently total correction with a homograft when 10 years of age. Over the years his homograft was degenerated and he had mild PS(pulmonary stenosis) and PR (pulmonary regurgitation),however he also developed severe aortic regurgitation and his aortic root and ascending aorta became aneurysmally dilated. At age 24 he underwent aortic valve replacement and a tube graft replacement of the ascending aorta. He had CAVB(complete atrioventricular block) and he is on DDD pacemaker since his first total correction.The CT angios show his anatomy prior to aortic valve replacement.

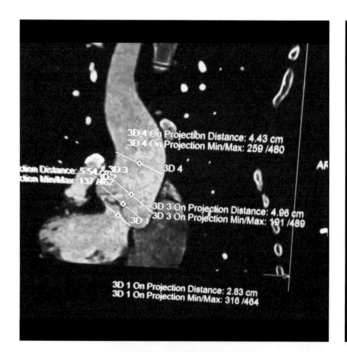
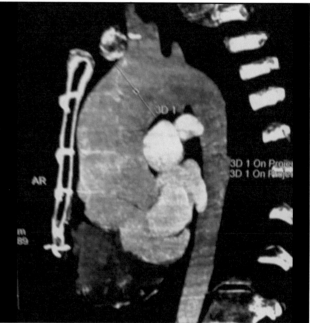

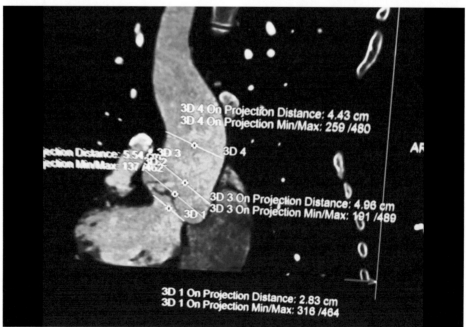

Figure 110: Note aneurysmally dilated sinus of Valsalva and the ascending aorta.

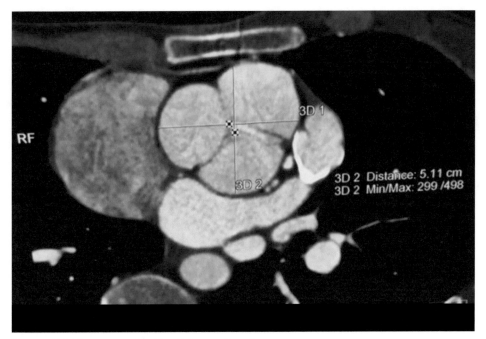

Figure 111: Note great details of the aortic valve cusps.

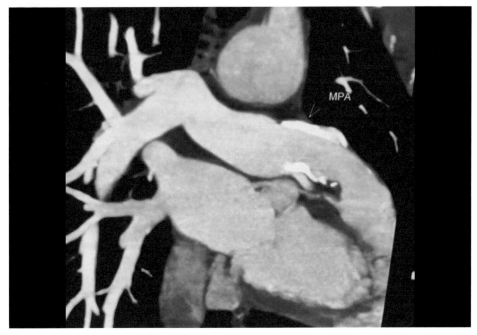

Figure 112: Note curved planar view of the RV (right ventricle), homograft and RPA(right pulmonary artery) below the cross section of the aorta and abovethe left ventricle and left atrium.

Case study:ME # 015

The patient is a 32-year-old male followed since 12 years of age. His CHD (congenital heart disease) was diagnosed at 2 years of age.The patient is emaciated, cyanotic with DOE (dyspnea on exertion).He has a sedentary job. He has recently married and has a 3-year-old healthy daughter by IVF(in vitro fertilization). He has massive cardiomegaly, primarily due to a huge RA(right atrium), secondary to massive TR(tricuspid regurgitation). His EKG shows first degree AV block, giant P-waves,due to right atrial hypertrophy and CRBBB (complete right bundle branch block).TV (tricuspid valve) attachment is normal and RV (right ventricle) is remarkable by multiple saccular spaces, and poor contraction.The patient has advanced form of RV noncompaction CMP (cardiomyopathy) with biventricular systo-diastolic dysfunction as studied by echocardiography and TD-mapping (tissue-Doppler mapping).The LV (left ventricular) dysfunction is less remarkable as compared to the RV(right ventricle). LV EF is 44% and RV EF is 37% by Simpson's method. LV does not show features of noncompaction CMP on echocardiography.RAVI (right atrial volume index) is 187.6 ml/m². Since 28 years of age he has developed PVCs (premature ventricular contractions), with bigeminy and some couplets.

Patient is on anticongestive therapy and receives periodic EECP (enhanced external counter-pulsation) therapy.

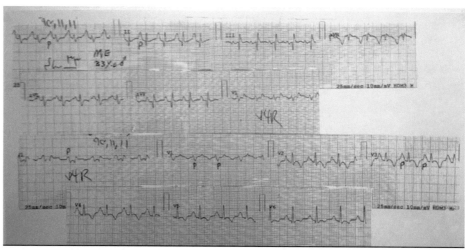

Figure 113: Note giant P waves in leads I,II,V4R, V1 and V3, due to massive right atrial enlargement .

Note CT angio frames:

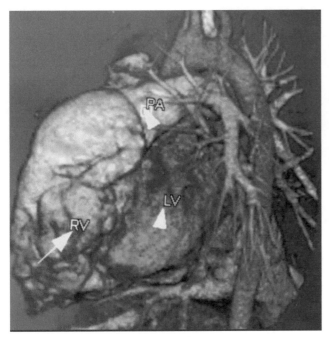

Figure 114: RV with saccular surface.

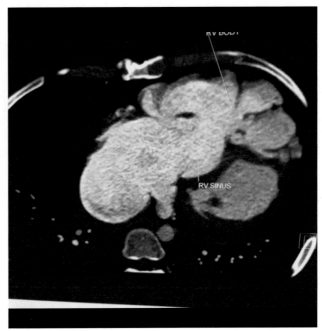

Figure 115: Giant RA filling 1/3 of the right hemithorax. Insertion of the TV cusps is shown by two dark notches between RA and RV inflow (sinus). The RV body is saccular.

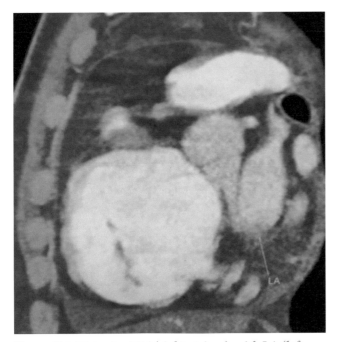

Figure 116: Note giant RA(right atrium), with LA (left atrium) posteriorly.

Case study:RSY # 255

Patient is a 3-month-old baby boy with TF (tetralogy of Fallot) and blue spells. CT angio was performed prior to a shunt. Note extremely narrow RVOT(right ventricular outflow tract), due to gross hypertrophy of the subpulmonary conus myocardium. This case is a perfect example of Van Praagh's description of the RV conus in TF as "a mighty midget", ie the conus is small but highly muscular.

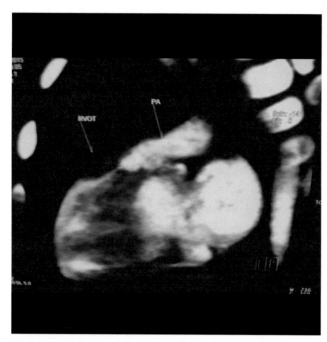

Figure 117: Note very narrow RVOT, due to gross hypertrophy of the RV infundibulum.

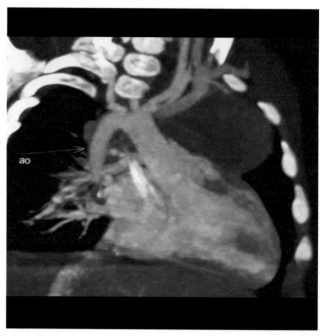

Figure 118: Note right aortic arch.

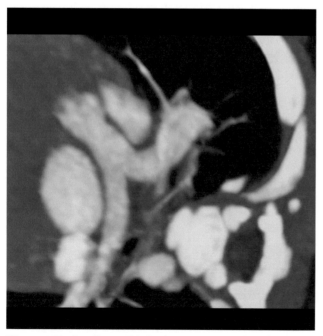

Figure 119: Confluent PA (pulmonary artery). Adequate size of MPA,LPA, and RPA

Case study:HK # 032

Patient presented at 75 days of age with DOE (dyspnea on exertion) and severe heart failure. EKG showed increased RV (right ventricular) pressure,LAH (left atrial hypertrophy) and BVH (biventricular hypertrophy) and diffuse ST-T changes. She had moderate mitral regurgitation.Tissue Doppler examination showed dysfunctional LVLW (left ventricular lateral wall),LVPW(left ventricular posterior wall), and IVS (ventricular septum). LAVI (left atrial volume index) was at the upper limit of normal. EF(ejection fraction) was 30% and FS (fractional shortening) was14.NT-proBNP was 36628pg/ml.A LR (left to right) continuous shunt was noted in the PA (pulmonary artery) sinus of Valsalva. Anomalous origin of the left coronary artery from the MPA (main pulmonary artery) was made. He was treated medically for heart failure and at 4 months of age, his heart failure though improved but persisted. EKG-gated CT angio was performed,which showed that MPA gave rise to the LMCA (left main coronary artery) from which LCX and LAD arose. RCA arose from the aorta,but it was huge in size and aneurysmal, causing LR shunt into the MPA. With fair control of heart failure the patient was referred to surgeon at 22 months of age for corrective surgery. Abnormal LCA was implanted on the aorta. The patient expired on the operating table.

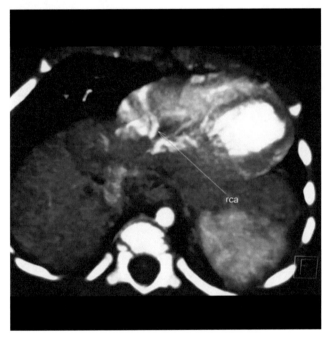 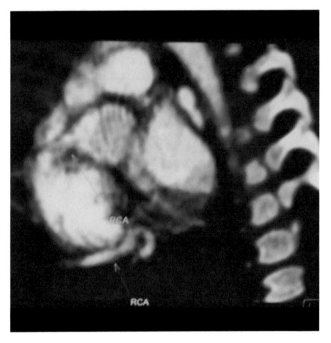

Figure 120: A huge RCA arising from the aorta.

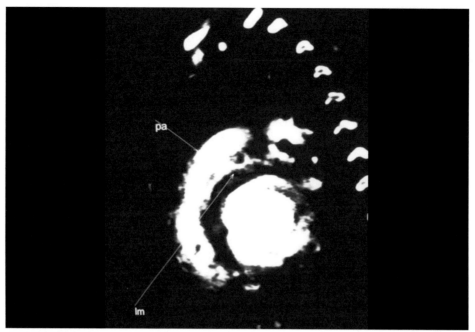

Figure 121: RV anterior and disc-shaped LV posteriorly. LMCA(left main coronary artery) arising from the main PA(pulmonary artery).

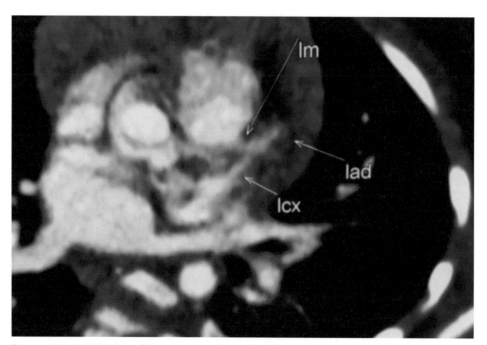

Figure 122: LM,LAD and LCX arising from the MPA.

Case study:MS # 034

The following CT angio frames are shown here for teaching purposes.The patient is an errratic case first seen at 11 months of age.Her 3rd visit was at 8 years of age and 4th visit was at 22 years of age. She had tricuspid atresia IB. She had undergone a right and subsequently a left BT(Blalock-Taussig) shunt. The third was a right Glenn shunt with ligation of the right BT shunt at 22 years of age.

At 22 years of age an unsuccessful attempt was made to divert IVC (inferior vena cava) flow to the left lung. But as this failed, the RPA (right pulmonary artery) was ligated and a central shunt was performed on the LPA(left pulmonary artery). A right lower lobe infarct developed due to CVP (central venous pressure) catheter. Also on CT angio, a diagnosis of extensive thrombosis in the brachicephalic vein, SVC(superior vena cava) and RPA(right pulmonary artery) was made.

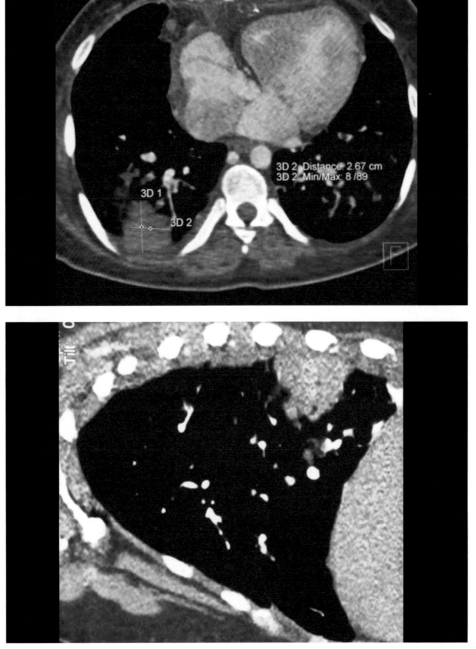

Figure 123: Right lower lobe infarct.This frame dated 22-Feb-1010.

The following frame was read as extensive brachiocephalic vein,SVC and RPA thrombosis.

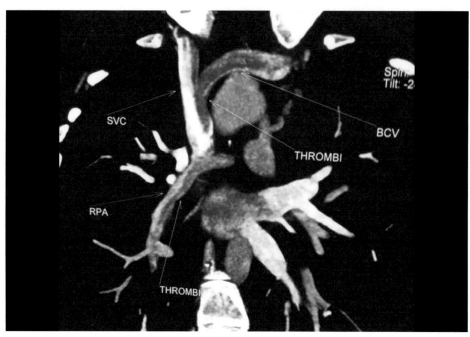

Figure 124: Note brachiocephaci vein(BCV) joining SVC, draining into the RPA (Rt
Glenn shunt).Extensive "thrombosis" noted in the RPA and SVC and BCV
(arrows).This frame dated 22-Feb-2010

Streptokinase therapy was carried out. However the following frame dated February 24, 2010,showed normal Glenn shunt and RPA. The interpretation of the previous frame was corrected, ie the image simulating thrombosis was due to laminar flow, not true venous thrombosis.

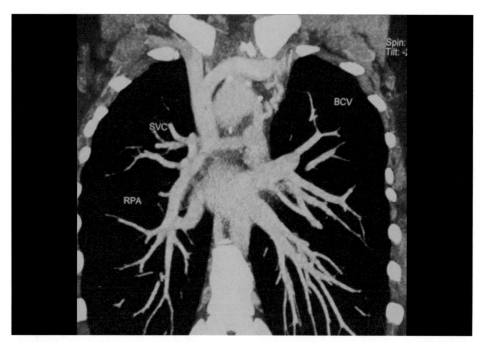

Figure 125: Note perfectly normal BCV,SVC and RPA. The previous diagnosis of
thrombosis was corrected,and re-interpreted as due to laminar flow. In all
cases of thromboemboli one should be aware of this phenomenon,leading
to an erroneous diagnosis of thrombosis or embolism.This frame dated
24-Feb-2010.

Case study: HD # 035

Patient is an 8-month-old baby girl who presented with severe heart failure, which probably began at the age of 4 months. She had severe LVH (left ventricular hypertrophy) with strain on EKG.On physical exam she had no femoral pulses. She had massive cardiomegaly and severe MR (mitral regurgitatgion) on echocardiography. A CT angio was performed to confirm the clinical diagnosis of the coarctation of the aorta.This study showed cardiac chamber enlargement. Normal coronaries and enlarged liver consistent with the clinical findings of heart failure.There was hypoplasia of a long segment of the abdominal aorta beginning at the level of the coeliac artery, with many collaterals,bypassing the area of hypoplasia.

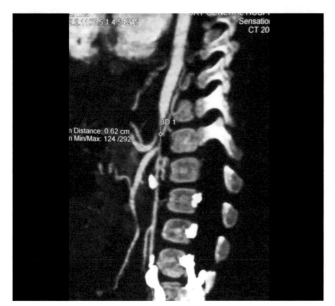
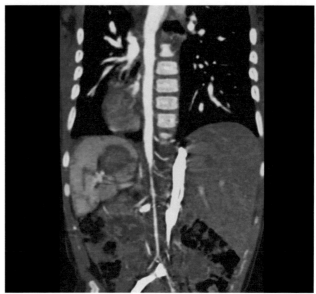

Figure 126: Hypoplasia of the descending aorta, beginning at the level of the coeliac artery.

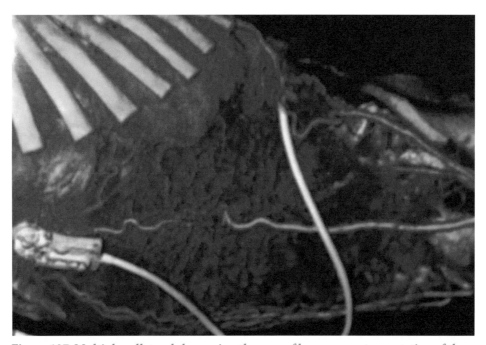

Figure 127: Multiple collaterals bypassing the area of long segment coarctation of the abdominal aorta.

Case study: HD # 081

A new entity:

Patient is a 6-year-old girl first diagnosed to have CHD(congenital heart disease) at 1 1/2 years of age. She has mild cyanosis.There is no murmur.Chest X-ray shows decreased PVM (pulmonary vascular markings) and PA (pulmonary artery) was small. EKG showed NSR (normal sinus rhthm),RAH(right atrial hypertrophy), QRS axis at -60 degrees. There were no RV(right ventricular) forces. She was catheterized elsewhere at 5 1/2 years of age.

Cath findings:There was an ASD (atrial septal defect) secundum type. TV (tricuspid valve) and RV(right ventricle) were small. RV (right ventricular) pressure was 25/0-8,PA(pulmonary artery) pressure was 20/8 mmHg.LV (left ventricular) pressure was 110/0-8,FA(femoral artery) pressure was 115/70 mmHg. Arterial PO2 45 mmHg, PCO2 25 mmHg, Sat 95%.Low PO2 due to RL shunting via ASD.

The diagnosis was agenesis of the RV apex and sinus, normal but small RV inflow and TV. The diagnosis thus was Hypoplastic RV syndrome, with RV sinus atresia. No intervention was recommended, because already the cardiac physiology was similar to a fenestrated Fontan, without any operation!

She was lost to follow-up and showed up again at 17 years of age, asking for marriage possibility. Again she was dusky and had clubbing of the finger-, and toe-nails. Pulse oximetry showed 82% saturation. EKG showed LAD (left axis deviation),RAH (right atrial hypertrophy),with ST-T changes in V5,V6 and aVL.

Echocardiography showed absent RV sinus. RVOT(right ventricular outflow tract) (conus) and PA were within normal limits. LV EF was 53 (Simpson) and 49 (M mode) FS 22. Cn 0.02 ;E deceleration time 170 msec.PA flow peak systolic 8 mmHg.There was no PR (pulmonary regurgitation).There was subclinical LV dysfunction similar to the first visit.A CT angio was performed.

Discussion: As there is a hypoplastic left heart syndrome (HLHS), there is also a hypoplastic right heart syndrome (HRHS). Similar to HLHS, which has a spectrum from complete form involving the MV(mitral valve), LV(left ventricle) and AO(aorta), ie mitral atresia alone, aortic atresia alone, or hypoplastic LV alone or in combination, I believe right heart atresia may also have several forms. As a matter of fact tricuspid atresia (TA) with its two types, ie type I with TGV and type II without TGV. Each one having three subtypes ie TA type IA with pulmonary atresia, type IB with pulmonary stenosis and type IC without pulmonary stenosis. Type II A with pulmonary atresia,Type IIB with pulmonary stenosis and type IIC without pulmonary stenosis,all should be looked at as one form of HRHS.

The heart we are describing is not tricuspid atresia in its classical form, however it represents a form of hypoplastic right heart syndrome.

To expand on the definition the hypoplastic right heart syndrome (HRHS), it may involve the tricuspid valve (TV),right ventricle (RV), or pulmonic valve (PV) isolated or in various combinations.

On one extreme there may be atresia of the entire right heart structures, complete form of hypoplastic right heart syndrome, typified by Goor's Heart. Or only the TV can be involved (tricuspid atresia and its variants, see above), or the PV could be involved alone, ie pulmonary atresia (with or without VSD) or the RV body could be hypoplastic.

We do know an entity of pulmonary atresia with intact ventricular septum. There are sinusoids from the coronary artery. Some 80 per cent show pulmonary valve atresia, but others present as critical pulmonary stenosis. The RA and LV are large and EKG shows LVH or predominatly LV forces and QRS axis is around

60 degrees, ie more to the left but rarely less than 0 degrees.LVH may be present as well. (The neonate with congenital heart disease. Richard D.Rowe and Ali Mehrizi. (pp p211-218) W.B.Saunders,Company, Philadelphia1968.).This entity should be looked at as one type in the spectrum of the hypoplastic right heart syndrome (HPHS).

The point is that, similar to the hypoplastic left heart syndrome, there exists a spectrum of hypoplastic right heart syndrome.Thus HLRH may present with or without VSD, and each type may be associated with pulmonary atresia,critical PS or no pulmonary stenosis,or tricuspid atresia, hypoplastic tricuspid valve or no tricuspid stenosis.The right ventricular ventricular sinus proper,may be totally absent or atretic,or be hypoplastic.

The case presented here is not yet known as an entity,but the major crieteria for its diagnosis are almost normal TV and pulmonic valves, but the RV sinus is atretic or absent. The anomaly must be accompanied with a stretched PFO or ASD to be compatible with life.

CT angio frames:

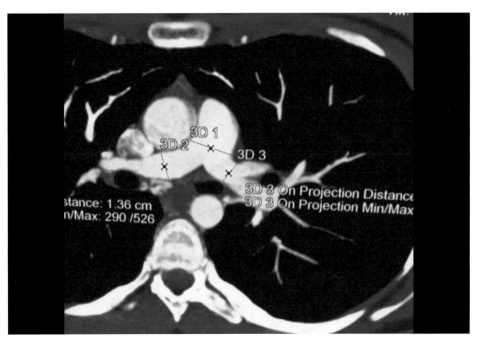

Figure 128: Normal main pulmonary artery(MPA) and branches. MPA 2.05 cm,right pulmonary artery(RPA) 1.36 cm and left pulmonary artery(LPA) 1.24 Cm in diameter.

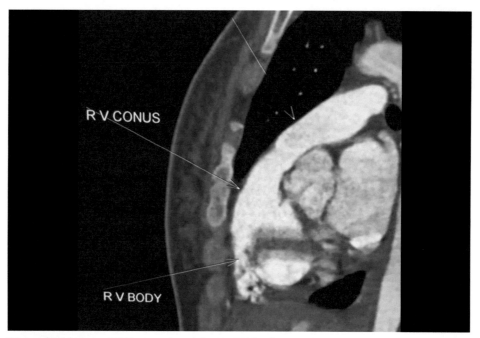

Figure 129: Normal RV conus,hypoplastic RV body or sinus.

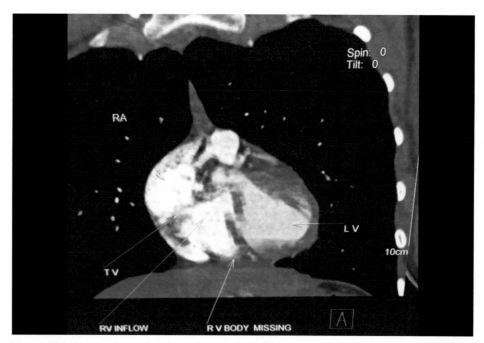

Figure 130: Note enlarged right atrium(RA) and left ventricle (LV). Right ventricular outflow tract is normal. Right ventricular (RV) sinus or body missing,ie atretic.

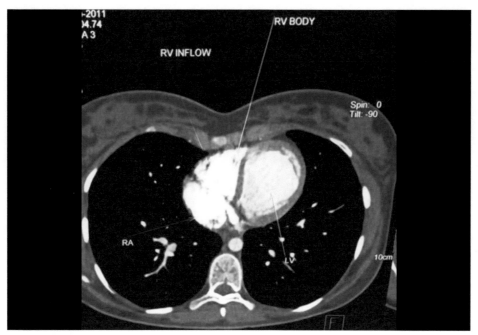

Figure 131: Note hypoplasia of the RV sinus.

For comparison normal RV is shown in three other patients.

HA a 5-month old girl:

Note normal RV in cross section and AP view. Note that RV fills out almost the entire anterior space of the image whereas LV fills out the posterior part.

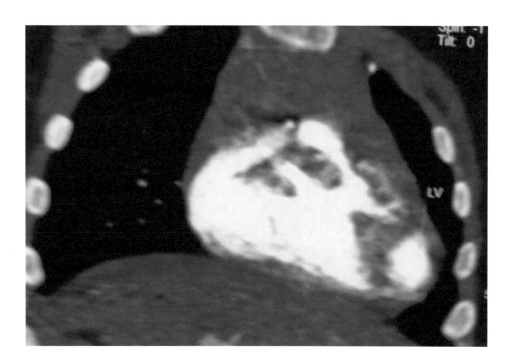

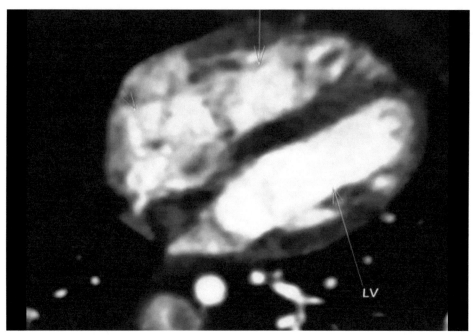

Figure 132: AP view to figure, horizontal section bottom figure, normal RV covers almost entirely the anterior part of the image.

Figures from a 25-year-old female. Note normal RV, inflow, sinus, outflow ie subpulmonary conus and normal MPA. RV fills out almost the entire cardiac silhouette anteriorly in frontal view. LV fills up almost the entire cardiac silhouette postertiorly in frontal view.

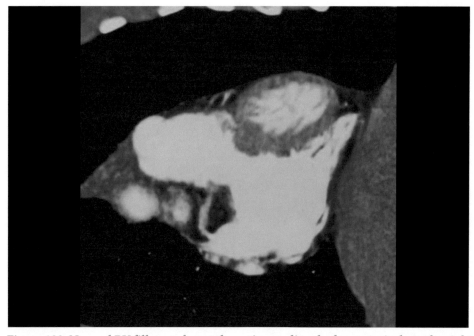

Figure 133: Normal RV fills out almost the entire cardiac shadow anteriorly to the right.

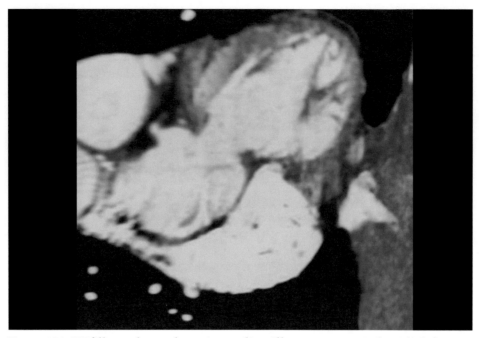

Figure 134: LV fills up almost the entire cardiac silhouette postertiorly to the left in coronal view.

To summarize:**Types of hypoplastic right heart syndrome:**

1-Tricuspid atresia (TA):

Tricuspid atresia has two types, with VSD and without VSD.However the type without VSD is very rare and when we talk about TA,we mean the type with VSD. This type has two types, Type I with normally related great vessels and type II with transposition (TGV). Each one has three subtypes:

IA: with pulmonary atresia,IB with PS(pulmonary stenosis),IC without PS.

IIA: with pulmonary atresia,IIB with PS(pulmonary stenosis),IIC without PS.

2-Pulmonary atresia with intact ventricular septum

3-Isolated hypoplasia or atresia of the RV sinus.(The case described above.)

The author has described two other new entities of congenital heart disease. See Epilogue for detailed description of these two anomalies.

Needless to stress that CT angio could be used to make the detailed anatomic description of these cases. The two cases in the Epilogue were detected before cardiovascular CT angio era.

Case study: MV #036

Patient is a 6-year-old boy who developed typical Kawasaki disease 1 month prior to the first visit.He was operated for appendicits during the acute phase of the disease. At the first visit he was anemic Hgb 8g/100 ml and his platelets were 559000/ml. His CT angio showed multiple aneurysms in the mid-portion of the RCA(right coronary artery). In the frames shown below aneurysm of the RCA, LCX(left circumflex) and LAD (left anterior descending) are demonstrated.

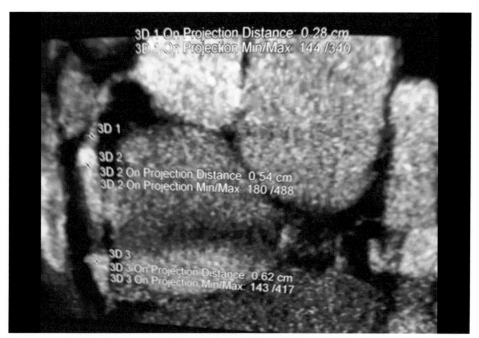

Figure 135: To the left of the frame note RCA originating from the aorta, with two aneurysms.RCA proper measures 0.28 cm in diameter.

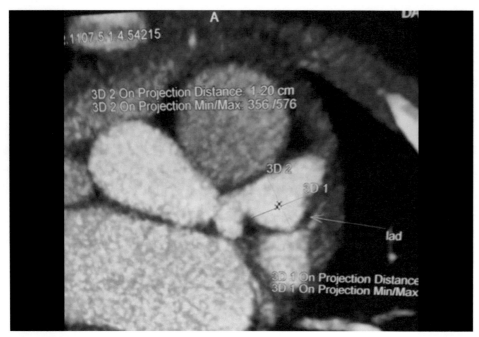

Figure 136: LAD aneurysm 1.2x1.16cm.

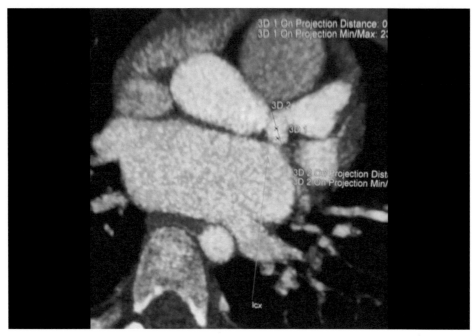

Figure 137: LCX aneurysm 0.63x0.95 cm

See references under Kawasaki disease.

Case study:MRR: #037

Patient is a 19-year old-boy followed since 2 years of age. He started with mild valvar PS (pulmonary stenosis) with peak gradient of 36 mmHg by Doppler method. The pulmonic valve was dysplastic.Over the years his PS became milder, at age 19 years his peak gradient was less than 10 mmHg, however gradually he developed enlarged MPA (main pulmonary artery) with turbulent flow. RVOT (right ventricular outflow tract) was 2.8 cm in diameter and pulmonary artery branches were were dilated.

A CT angio was performed. RVOT was within normal limits. However MPA(main pulmonary artery) and proximal portion of both RPA (right pulmonary artery) and LPA(left pulmonary artery) were aneurysmally dilated. His EKG intially showed mild RVH(right ventricular hypertrophy), however later on it has been within normal limits.He is asymptomatic and has been advised against competitive sports.

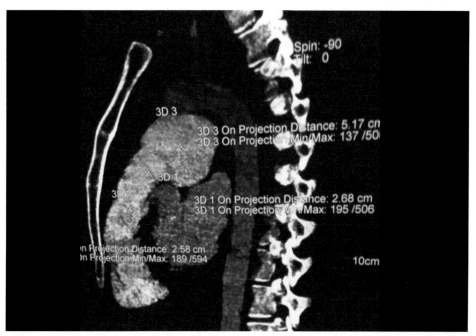

Figure 138: Aneurysmally dilated MPA.

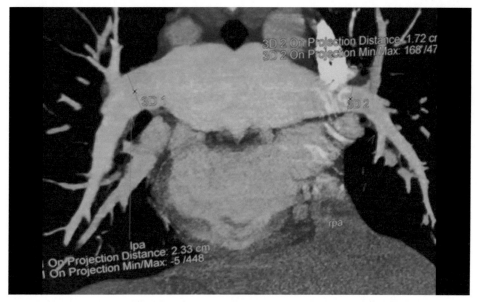

Figure 139: Aneurysmally dilated proximal RPA and LPA, but peripheral branches are wnl.

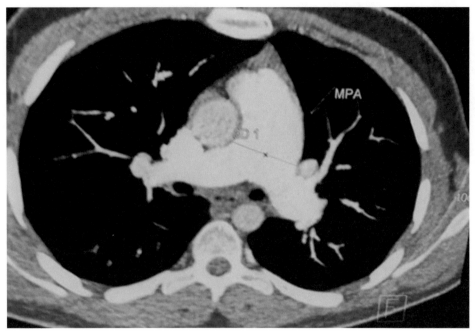

Figure 140: MPA aneursymally dilated 3.96 cm in diameter.

Case study: IH #049

Patient is a 19-year-old male first seen at 7 months of age with a diagnosis of tricuspid atresia (TA) type IIC, ie with dTGV(transposition of the great vessels) and no PS (pulmonary stenosis). He had increased PA (pulmonary artery) flow and heart failure. PA banding was performed at 18 months of age,with PG(peak gradient) of 50 mmHg postoperatively.At 4 years of age PAB(pulmonary artery band) gradient was 75 mmHg and there was no MR(mitral regurgitation).At 8 yrs of age PAB peak gradient was 80 mmHg. Patient was unsuitable for Fontan operation. LV(left ventricle) was quite large and patient was cyanotic. At 10 years of age patient developed hepatitis B. Followeing recovery,not being suitable for Fontan procedure, because of LV systolic and diastolic dysfunction, and a PAB,peak gradient of 106 mmHg, a shunt was recommended. Parents decided to go abroad for Fontan operation.The patient did not show up for periodic check-ups.

He returned at 12 yrs of age and a right BT shunt was performed.Catheterized at 15 years of age. VSD(ventricular septal defect) was restrictive with LV pressure 200 mmHg and aorta 120 mmHg, PA pressure wa 55/30 mmHg.

The patient had a tonsillectomy and adenoidectomy for severe upper respiratory tract obstruction at 15 yrs of age.

At 16 years of age a right central shunt was performed to relieve hypoxia. Postoperatively he developed heart failure, which intensified gradually with development of severe MR(mitral regurgitation).

Being in desperate shape, enlargement of the VSD and mitral valve replacement were recommended. However several months later,still undecided regarding operation, the patient expired with severe heart failure and CNS damage.

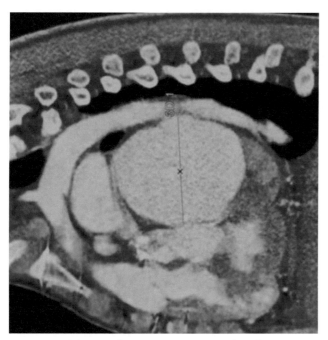

Figure 141: Tricuspid atresia IIC; note PA band on posterior PA and anterior Aorta.

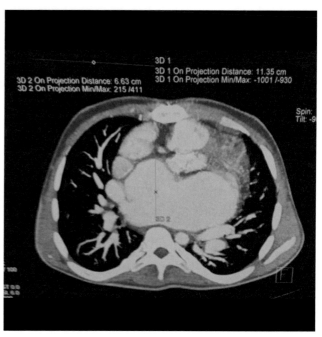

Figure 143: Massive LA enlargement due to severe MR.

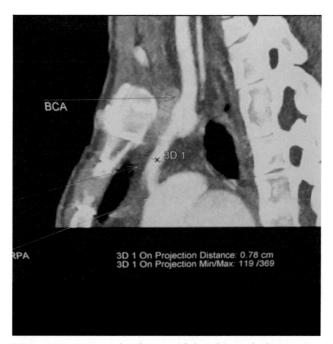

Figure 142: Note right shunt with brachiocephalic artery on top and RPA at bottom receiving the shunt.

Case study: ASF #060

Patient is a 30-year-old male who was first seen at 7 years of age with severe aortic valvar stenosis (AS), for which he had been operated elsewhere at 7 months of age. He was catheterized elsewhere and was found to have 30 mmHg residual aortic stenosis and mild AR (aortic regurgitation).

At 8 years of age he had 60 mmHg peak gradient across the aortic valve and he had moderate AR with heart failure. Aortic valve replacement was recommended, but patient did not follow instruction, and showed up at 13 years of age with severe AR and AS. Aortic valve replacement was again recommended. The patient disappeared and showed up again at 16 years of age.AS peak gradient was 90 mmHg and there was severe AR and moderate MR (mitral regurgitation). He had aortic valve replacement St Judes' valve #23. At 19 years of age he had moderate MR. His MR gradually improved with anticongestive treatment and a normally functioning prosthetic aortic valve. At 25 years of age he had frequent unifocal PVC's. He became an architect and married.

Though asymptomatic at 28 years of age, his EKG showed negative T waves in I,II,aVL,V4-V6.

He gradually became obese and at 30 years he presented with anginal pain and DOE (dyspnea on exertion). He had also developed presyncope while swimming. With SMVET (submaximal voluntary exercise test) he had syncope at 10.4 METs, HR 144/min. but no further EKG changes. TTT (tilt table test) was negative.

He had MRI stress test which showed normal myocardial perfusion,and no ischemia was induced.

Simultaneous coronary CT angio showed a dilated ascending aorta. This study showed normal coronaries with no obstruction, however RCA (right coronary artery) had a more medial take-off, as compared to normal. The presumptive diagnosis for presyncopal state and anginal pains with effort is the compression of the RCA between the aorta and RVOT. Despite this CT angio diagnosis, microvessel coronary artery disease could also be the reason for ischemic symptoms.

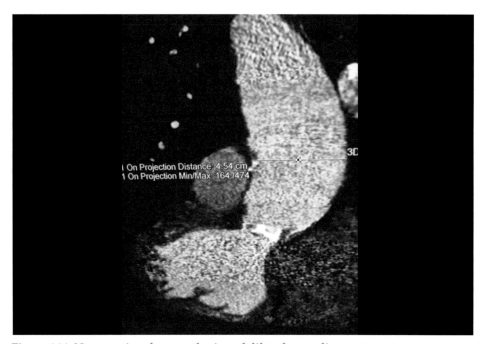

Figure 144: Note aortic valve prosthesis and dilated ascending aorta.

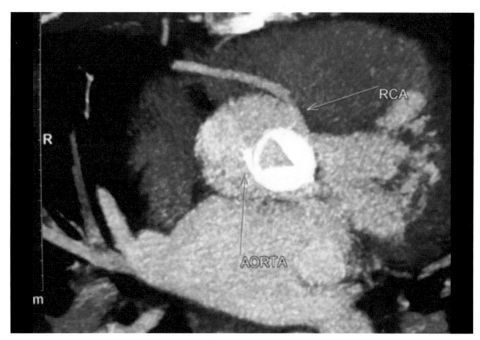

Figure 145: Note more medial take-off of the RCA coursing between the aortic root and RVOT.

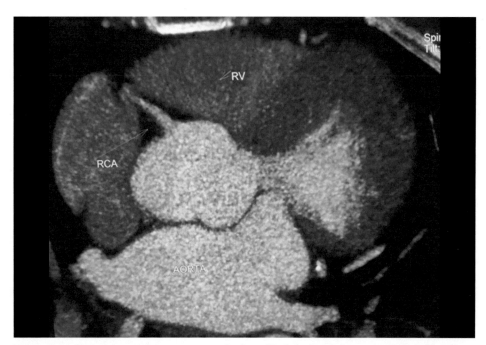

Figure 146: For comparison note normal take-off of the RCA from another patient.

Case study:AA #050

Patient is a 20-year-old male first seen at 24 days of age with diagnosis of TF (tetralogy of Fallot). At 2 1/2 years of age he weighed 9 kg and was cyanotic. He had a left 5-mm Goretex shunt.At 5 1/2 years of age he underwent total correction with VSD (ventricular septal defect) closure and transannular RVOT(right ventricular outflow tract) patch.A moderate residual VSD with VSD patch aneurysm bulging into the RVOT was present. On cardiac catheterization QP/QS was 2.5 /1, with RPA(right pulmonary artery),LPA(left pulmonary artery) origin stenosis. Revision was recommended at 6 years of age. Presently the patient has DOE (dyspnea on exertion),and he has RVOT patch aneurysm, plus moderate to severe PR (pulmonary regurgitation). Reoperation (RVOT repair and pulmonary valve replacement) was recommended based on echocardiographic and CT angio findings.

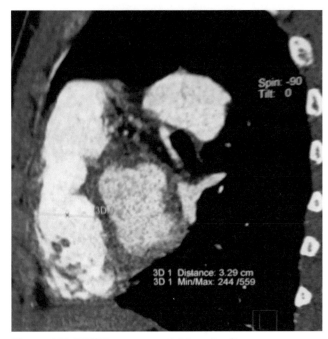 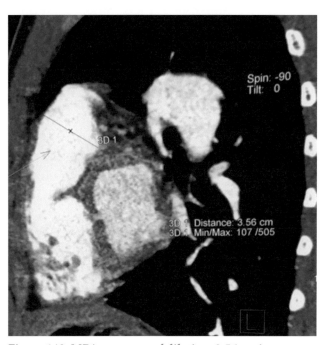

Figure 147: RVOT aneurysm,3.29 cm in diameter.

Figure 148: MPA aneurysmal dilation, 3.56 cm in diameter.

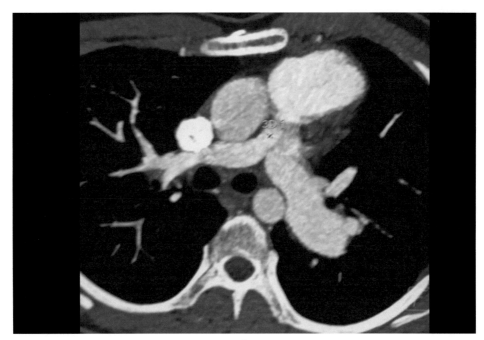

Figure 149: LPA origin stenosis 0.93 cm in diameter.

The following frames belong a to a 27-year-old girl whose tetralogy of Fallot was corrected at 6 years of age. This CT angio was performed before pulmonic valve replacement and RVOT aneurysm repair.

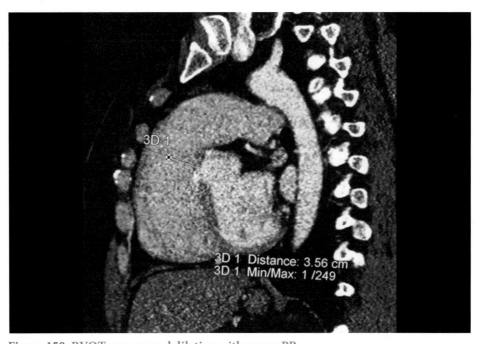

Figure 150: RVOT aneurysmal dilation with severe PR.

Case study: SA #039

The power of CT angiography in delineating pulmonary artery system is exemplified by this case. The patient a 10-yr-old female with tetralogy of Fallot and pulmonary atresia was found on cardiac catheterization to have one large collateral feeding the entire right lung and two collaterals were noted on the left side. The collaterals on the left were ligated and a shunt implanted on the "LPA".

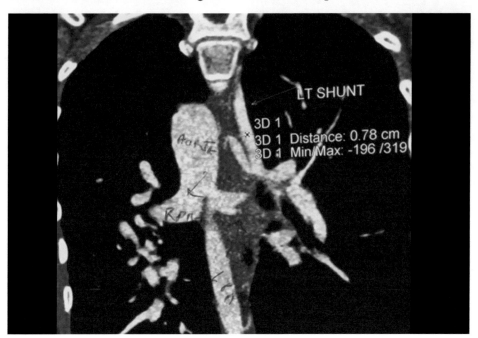

Figure 151: Note right aortic arch. Both lungs receive a large collateral at the level of T7. On a previous operation "LPA" (ie the left collateral was ligated and a left central shunt implanted on the "LPA", which is a collateral.

97

Case study: BX # 043

This patient was first seen at 12 days of age with TF (tetralogy of Fallot) and pulmonary atresia. A left shunt was performed at 2 months of age. This CT angio study is prior to total correction.

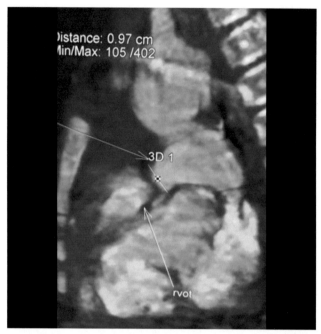

Figure 152: TF with pulmonary atresia.

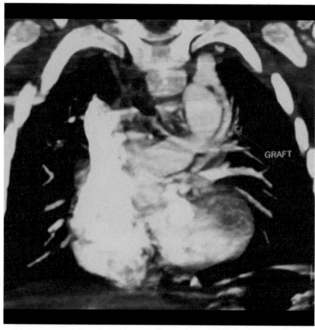

Figure 153: Shunt on the LPA.

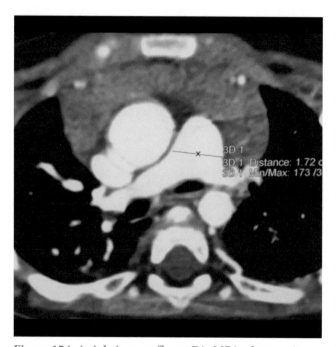

Figure 154: Axial view confluent PA, MPA adequate in size 1.72 cm.

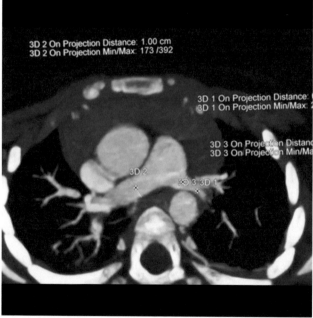

Figure 155: RPA 1 cm in diameter, LPA hypoplastic 0.29-0.34 cm in diameter.

Case study: MTS #044

Patient is a 5.5- year-old boy who presented first at 9 months of age with elfine facies, typical of infantile hypercalcemia or William's syndrome. He had supravalvar aortic stenosis and bilateral small LPA (left pulmonary artery) and RPA (right pulmonary artery).A CT angio was performed because Doppler showed 40 mmHg peak systolic gradient above the aortic valve.

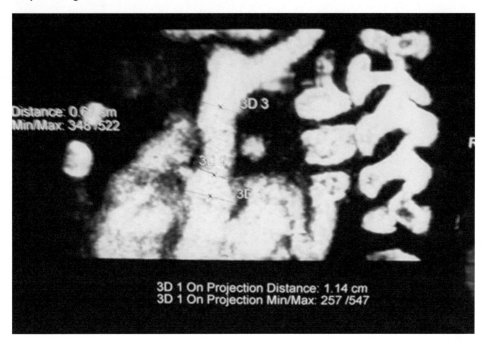

Figure 156: Initial CT angio 6 months preop: Aortic diameter 1.14 cm, proximal end of stenosis 0.67 cm, distal end of the stenosis 0.82 cm.

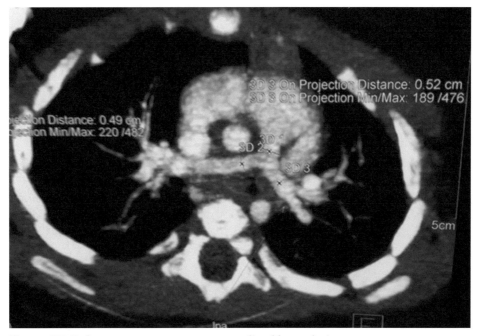

Figure 157: Pulmonary artery system,generalized hypoplasia.

Cardiac catheterization prior to surgical repair at 2 years of age showed funnel-shaped supravalvar tubular stenosis with LV(left ventricular) pressure 150/0-9 mmHg, distal aorta 67/58(63) mmHg.There was generalized hypoplasia of the pulmonary artery system, with RV(right ventricle) 52/0-6mmHg, MPA(main pulmonary artery) 52/13(mean 30)mmHg and LPA (left pulmonary artery) 25/15 mmHg.

Post-surgical repair at 4 years of age.

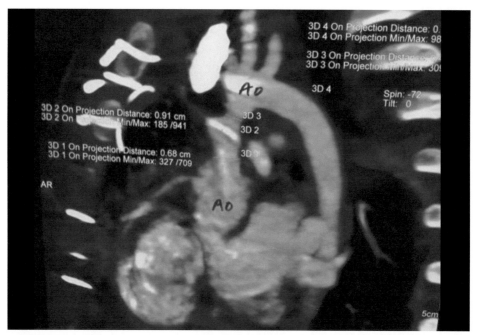

Figure 158: Postop CT angio shows upward shifting of the area of obstruction with 54 mmHg peak gradient by Doppler.

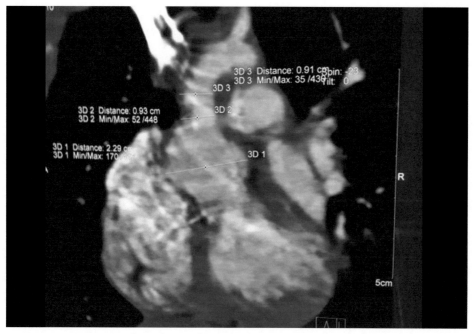

Figure 159: At 4 years of age the patch area is dilated 2.29 cm, with distal end of the ascending aorta 0.93 cm in diameter.Peak systolic gradient by Doppler 55 mmHg.

See references under aortic stenosis.

Case study: YK #065

Patient is a 29-year-old male followed since 5 years of age. Congenital heart disease was diagnosed at 4 years of age.He had moderate MR (mitral regurgitation) treated with digoxin. AR(aortic regurgitation) was first noted at 8 years of age. Because of severe AR the aortic valve was replaced and mitral valve was repaired at 14 years of age.He did fine but his MR gradually increased. By 19 years of age he had moderate MR. He had signs of Marfan's syndrome. He was last seen at 25 years of age with moderate MR. He was lost to follow-up and showed up again at 29 years of age with SOB (shortness of breath), and DOE (dyspnea on exertion). He also had episodes of transient ischemic attacks.Valve clicks were muffled. On echocardiography he had severe MR and very limited aortic valve motion and there was almost no flow across the valve orifice.

Emergency AOVR(aortic valve replacement) (ONX 27), aortic tube graft #20,Benthal operation,for repair of the aneurysmal ascending aorta, and MVR (mitral valve replacement)(ONX 29) were performed.CABG (coronary artery bypass graft) was needed for impingement of the valves on the RCA (right coronary artery). A VVI pacemaker was necesssary for CAVB (complete atrioventricular block).The pacemaker was subsequently changed to DDD pacemaker.

Pathology report of the aortic wall showed cystic medial degeneration consistent with Marfan's syndrome.

At last exam at 29 years of age, the patient is asymptomatic, prior going to the USA for Neurophysics PhD course. MV peak gradient 9-12 mmHg. AOV functioning well with minimal anterior leak.Pacemaker function normal.There was no heart failure. Discharge medications were warfarin and propranolol.

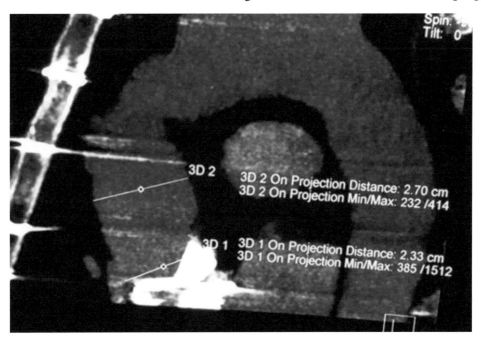

Figure 160: AO valve replaced.Note dilated ascending aorta.

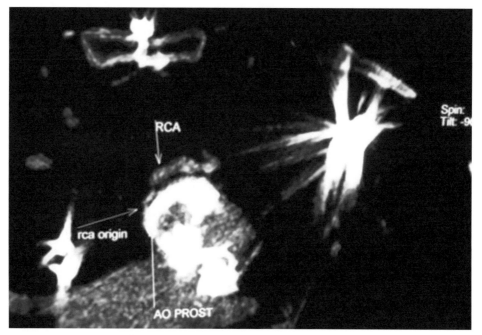

Figure 161: Note mitral valve prosthesis to the right of the frame. RCA impingement by the aortic valve.

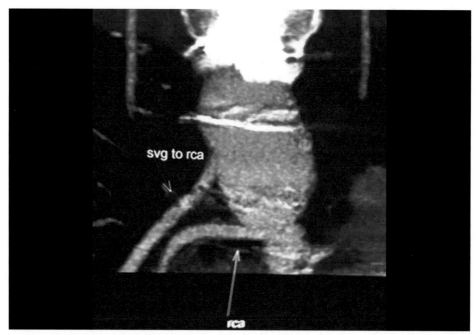

Figure 162: CABG on the RCA.

Case study:RJ #045

Patient is a 14-year-old male first seen at 7 months of age with EFE (endocardial fibroelastosis) vs acquired CMP(cardiomyopathy), coarctation of the aorta, and bicuspid aortic valve. He underwent total correction of discrete coarctation. At 9 months of age he had no residual coarctation and no aortic stenosis.At 15 months of age there was no LV (left ventricular) dysfunction and coarctation site was normal with no stenosis. He was lost to follow-up, and showed up again at 14 years of age. He was obese. There was no aortic stenosis. Coarctation of the aorta site showed 24-31 mmHg peak gradient by Doppler, however his BP was normal and the femoral pulses were normal in amplitude. EKG was within normal limits.

A CT angio was performed.This study showed AAO (ascending aorta)1.97 cm in diameter. The narrowest diameter,proximal isthmus was 0.99 cm and distal part 1.98 cm in diameter. The patient was advised to keep the weight within normal range, and be punctual on follow-up visits.

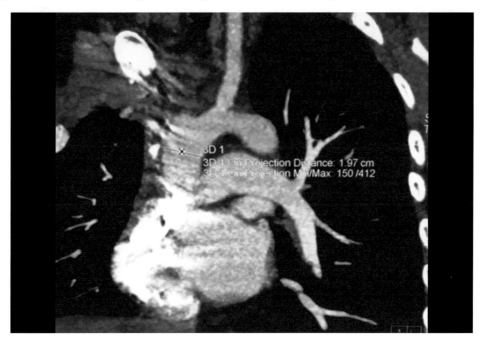

Figure 163: Dilated ascending aorta.

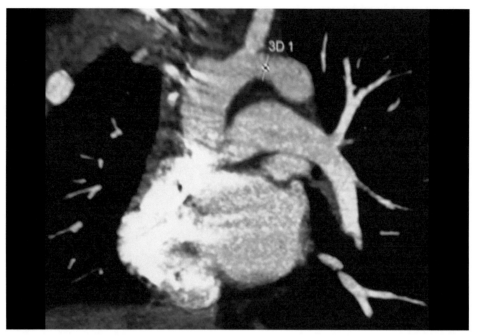

Figure 164: Proximal aortic isthmus 0.99 cm in diameter.

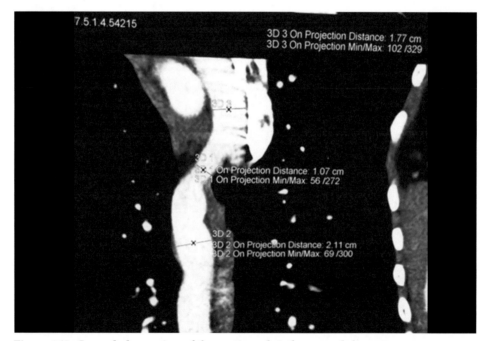

Figure 165: Curved planar view of the aortic arch, isthmus and thoracic aorta, measuring 1.77, 1.07 and 2.11 cm in diameter respectively.

See References, Baumgartner et al. under coarctation of the aorta.

Case study:SB #046

Patient was first seen at the age of 3 years.She had DORV(double outlet ventricle) without TGV(transposition of the great vessels) and moderate PS (pulmonary stenosis). She underwent total correction in England, with transannular patch and VSD (ventricular septal defect) closure. Postoperatively at 7 years of age, she had heart failure with mild PS (pulmonary stenosis) and moderate PR (pulmonary regurgitation).RVOT was aneurysmal. A small residual VSD closed spontaneously at 11 years of age.At 14 years of age RVOT aneurysm measured 3.50 cm in diameter, with mild PS and moderate PR 8 mmHg PG by Doppler.

At 24 years of age she had severe PR,RVOT was 3.77 cm in diameter.She was studied with CT angio. Based on clinical findings supported by CT angio, elective repair of the RVOT and PVR (pulmonary valve replacement) was recommended anticipating marriage, pregnancy and delivery. Patient disappeared following this study.

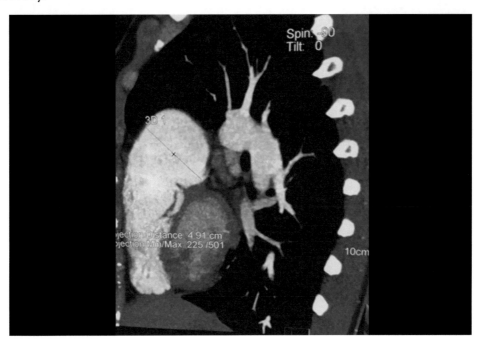

Figure 166: Gross RVOT aneurysm.

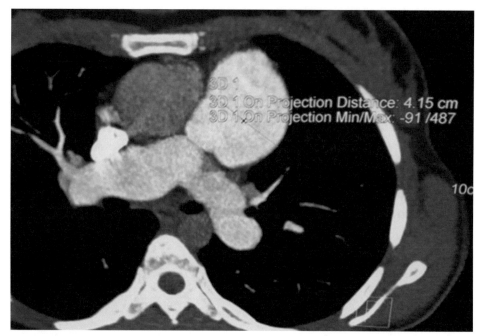

Figure 167: RVOT and MPA aneurysmal dilation.

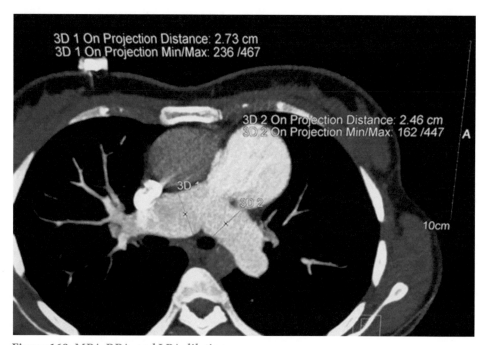

Figure 168: MPA,RPA, and LPA dilation.

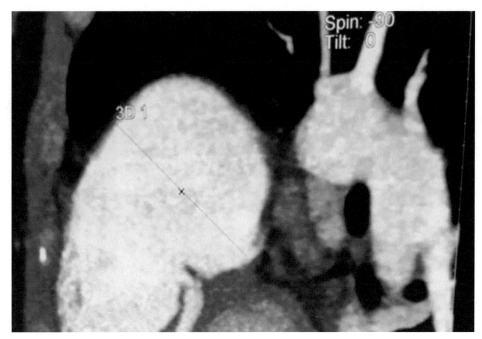

Figure 169: Aneurysmal dilation of the RVOT and MPA,4.91 cm in diameter.

Case study:HB #053

Patient is a 7-year-old boy first seen at 5 months of age.He was in heart failure and had low atrial rhythm on EKG.He had situs inversus, with meso-,or levocardia, d-TGV,VSD(ventricular septal defect) in ECD(endocardial cushion) position, severe PS (pulmonary stenosis) and ?PAPVD (partial anomalous pulmonary venous drainage) on echocardiography.With diagnosis of Ivemark syndrome he had a CT angio at the age of 2 1/2 years.

CT angio revealed situs inversus, meso-, or levocardia. Two SVC's were present,with RSVC draining into the LA, pulmonary venous return was normal. A large cushion type VSD was present. PS and subvalvar outflow tract obstruction were present plus d-TGV, and right aortic arch.

At 5 years of age he underwent total correction.

Patient had heart failure with moderate TR (tricuspid regurgitation) postoperatively.TR continues with mild RV (right ventricular) dysfunction.

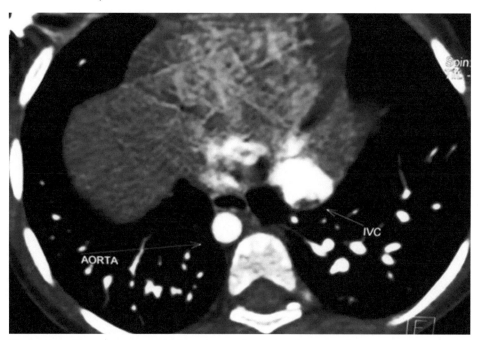

Figure 170: Situs inversus with the aorta to the right of spine and IVC anteriorly to the left.

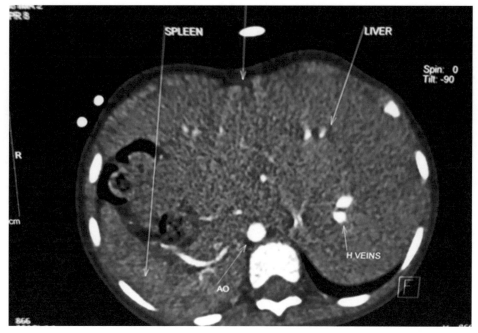

Figure 171: Situs inversus with liver and hepatic vein to the left and aorta to the right.

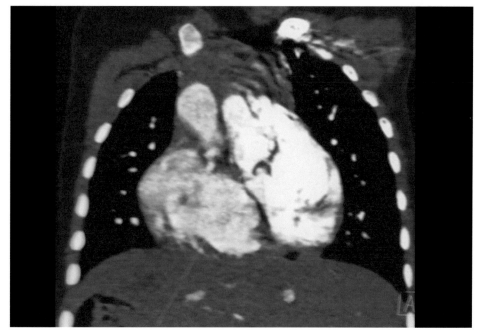

Figure 172: Situs inversus, mesocardia or levocardia, note conus under the aortic valve to the right and MPA (main pulmonary artery) to the left.So:IDD.

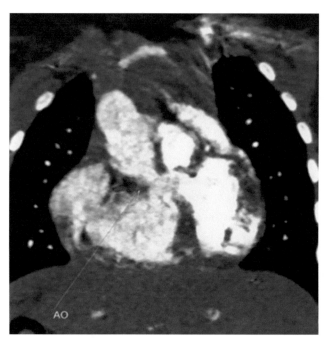

Figure 173: Note liver on the left, situs inversus, heart in the middle or left, meso-, or levocardia, ie Ivemark syndrome. Conus under the right sided aorta (red arrow), so RV on the right, aorta originating from the RV, large cushion type VSD,pulmonic valve to the left of the aorta, so D-loop ventricles, and d-loop great vessels,ie IDD.

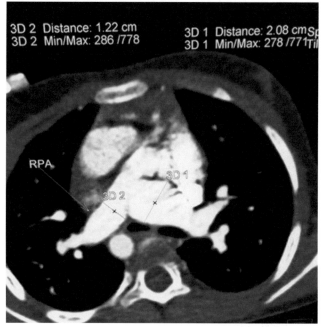

Figure 175: Confluent PA system,with dilated LPA 2.08 cm in diameter.

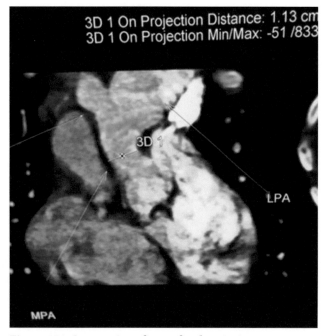

Figure 174: See previous figure for description.

Case study: HA # 062

Patient is a 3-month-old girl with cystinuria and renal calculi who presented with heart failure. She had complete endocardial cushion defect,with mitral and tricuspid regurgitation and heart failure.

CT angio shows enlarged heart and situs solitus. The large cushion defect is noted in the last frame.

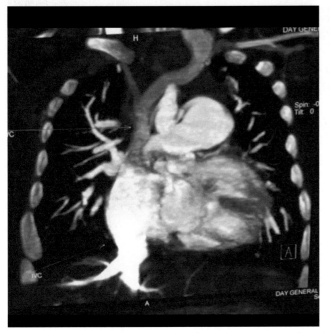 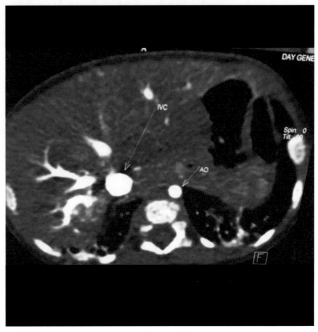

Figure 176: Situs solitus, note SVC (superior vena cava) and IVC(inferior vena cava) in the top figure draining into the right-sided RA(right atrium).In bottom figure with liver on the right,note aorta to the left and IVC to the right.

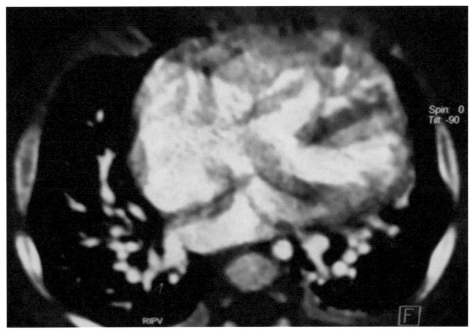

Figure 177: Large endocardial cushion defect type VSD.LV (left ventricle) below,RV (right ventricle) on top right of the figure. Mitral valve(MV) and tricuspid valve(TV) clefts were noted on echocardiography.

Case study: MPR # 068

The following study belongs to an 8-month-old boy with short segment coarctation of the aorta,and a high muscular VSD (ventricular septal defect) with heart failure.

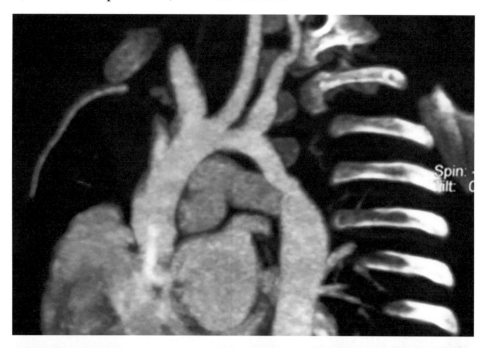

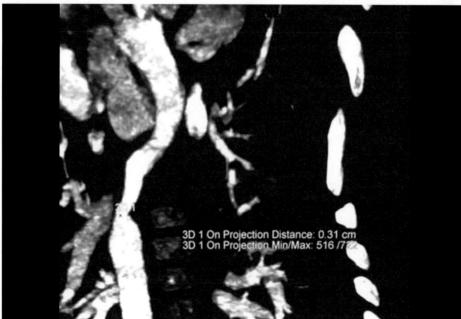

Figure 178: Short segmental coarctation of the aorta with narrowest diameter of 0.31 cm.The ascending aorta is 0.90 cm and the thoracic aorta is 0.97 cm in diameter.

Case study: ZX # 070

Patients with surgically corrected coarctation of the aorta may develop recoarctation due to sluggish growth of the narrow operated segment of the aortic isthmus. The case presented here serves as a good example, how spurious recoarctation could be diagnosed from true recoarctation of the aorta.

The patient was first seen at 20 days of age with gross LVH(left ventricular septal defect), coarctation of the aorta (peak gradient by Doppler 60 mmHg) and PDA(patent ductus arteriosus). She underwent surgical repair of the coarctation at 22 days of age with left subclavian flap. Over the years she improved remarkably with resolution of her severe LVH (left ventricular hypertrophy). Ever since operation she has had a weak left brachial pulse, normal blood pressure in the right arm, and palpable bilateral femoral pulses of good amplitude. However a peak gradient of 45-48 mm Hg by Doppler was present in the descending aorta. Before schooling at 6 1/2 years of age she had a CT-angio study which showed good repair. A spurious gradient is frequently encountered during echo-Doppler study, in patients who have undergone correction. The grdient is due to turbulent flow generated by an aortic isthmus with variable diameters in its various segments.

See the paper by Baumgartner under the references for coarctation of the aorta.

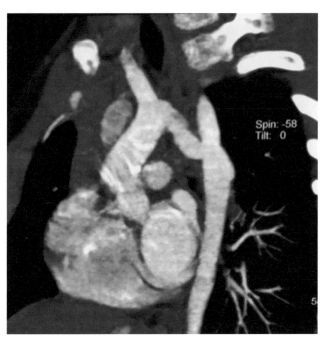

Figure 179: Note aortic arch anatomy, embryologically originating from different parts of the branchial system, with various lengths and diameters.This frame is post-total correction of the aorta in infancy.

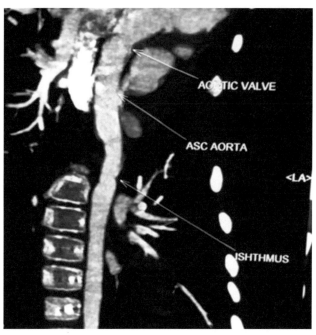

Figure 180: In this curved planar view of the aortic arch and upper thoracic aorta,adequacy of the lumen is best demonstrated.

Various diameters of different segments of the aortic isthmus,give rise to turbulence and spurious pressure gradient by Doppler study.

Case study: FM # 071

Patient is a 25-year-old male followed since 8 years of age with diagnosis of situs solitus, dextrocardia, VSD(ventricular septal defect), valvar and subvalvar PS (pulmonary stenosis),L-loop, LTGV. PA arising from the right sided LV, aorta arising from the left-sided LV. He underwent total correction at 16 years of age, with a homograft for MPA (main pulmonary artery). At 25 years of age he has moderate TR (tricuspid regurgitation). This CT angio was performed to evaluate PA (pulmonary artery) and the homograft not accessible by echocardiography.

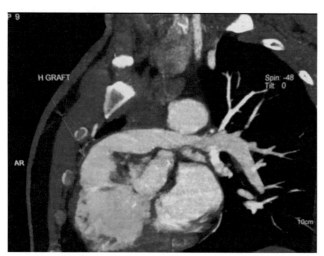

Figure 181: Situs solitus, liver right-sided. Dextrocardia. RV (right ventricle) on the right, LV (left ventricle) on the left. Homograft connecting RV to the PA(pulmonary artery), in good shape.

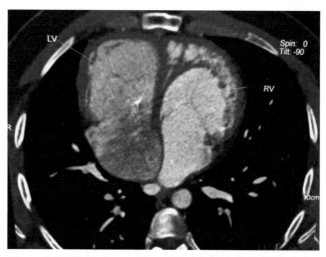

Figure 183: Note situs solitus, RA (right atrium) is right sided connecting to the right sided LV(left ventricle), LA(left atrium) left sided connecting to the left sided RV (right ventricle), ie L-TGV. Presently the tricuspid valve shows moderate regurgitataion because RV is maintaining the systemic circulation.

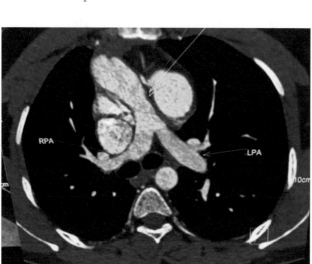

Figure 182: Noncalcified homograft, and PA (pulmonary arterial) branches.

Case study: MR # 072

Patient is a 4-month-old baby boy,who was referred for heart failure.His EKG showed extreme RVH (right ventricular hypertrophy) and he had cor bovinum on chest X-ray. NT-proBNP was 33,354 pg/ml. A CT angio was performed.

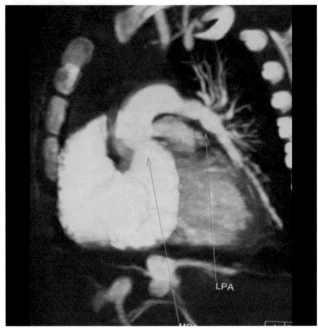

Figure 184: LPA (left pulmonary artery) originating from MPA(main pulmonary artery).

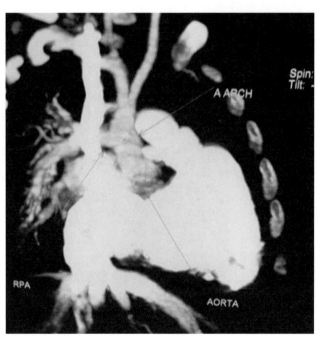

Figure 186: Ascending aorta giving rise to the RPA (right pulmonary artery). Hemitruncus.

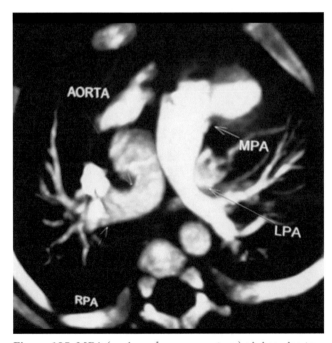

Figure 185: MPA (main pulmonary artery) giving rise to the LPA (left pulmonary artery).

Case study: EAK # 076

Patient is a 24 -year-old girl who was first seen at 14 months of age with diagnosis of LTGV(L transposition of the great vessels),VSD (ventricular septal defect), pulmonary vascular obstructive disease with pulmnary hypertension. She had a pulmonary artery banding shortly before the first visit elsewhere. Over the years she was followed with medical therapy. She began to have SOB(shortness of breath) and DOE (dyspnea on exertion) and increasing cyanosis worsening at 12 years of age.A CT angio was performed at 21 years of age.

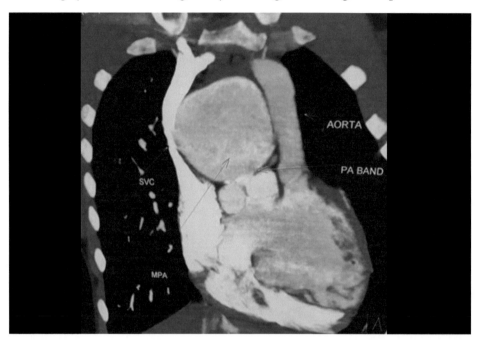

Figure 187: Situs solitus, note L-loop Ao (aorta) and PA(pulmonary artery), ie aorta to the left and PA to the right;aneurysmal dilation of the MPA(main pulmonary artery), and a tight PA band.

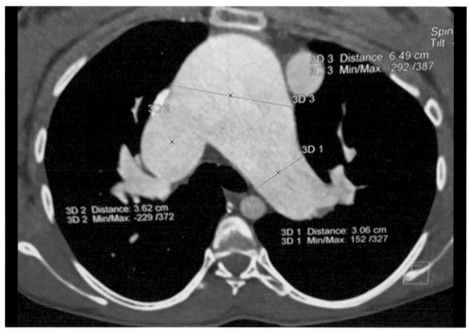

Figure 188: Aneurysmal dilation of the MPA(main pulmonary artery),LPA(left pulmonary artery) and RPA(right pulmonary artery) secondary to pulmonary vascular obstructive disease (due to Eisenmenger).

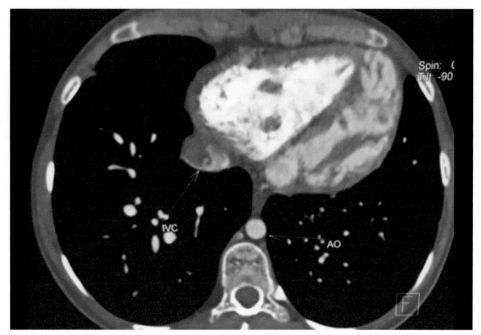

Figure 189: Note anterior ventricle with 2 papillary muscles (LV), and heavily trabeculated posterior ventricle (RV), ie L-TGV.

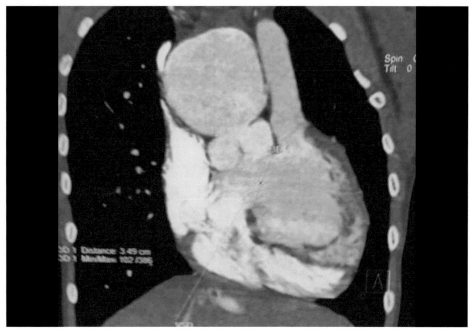

Figure 190: Aorta to the left of MPA(main pulmonary artery),ie LTGV in situ solitus, large VSD (ventricular septal defect) with the LV (left ventricle) feeding the PA(pulmonary artery) and RV(right ventricle) feeding the aorta.PA band and aneurysmal MPA on top left.

Case study: KR #078

Patient is a 16-year-old male followed since 4 years of age. He had DORV(double outlet right ventricle) with TGV (transposition of the great vessels),ie Taussig-Bing anomaly.He underwent a left Goretex shunt at 6 years of age.Subsequently he underwent a Rastelli procedure with a valved-Contegra-conduit for the MPA (main pulmonary artery) and pulmonary valve.He had anomalous origin of the left main coronary artery.At 9 year of age because of a residual VSD (ventricular septal defect) and subpulmonary stenosis,he underwent repeat operation, and a bovine xenograft was used this time for the pulmonary artery.Two years later the xenograft was degenerated with 40 mmHg peak systolic gradient and moderate TR (tricuspid regurgitation) 52 mmHg peak gradient.

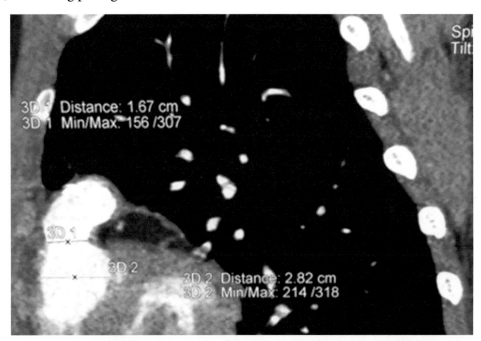

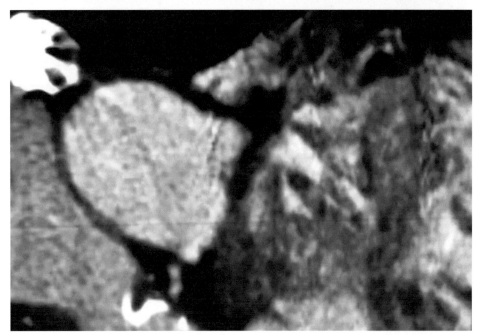

Figure 191: Dilated RVOT (right ventricular outflow tract) and calcified homograft wall.

Case study: PN #087

Patient is a 10-year-old girl who underwent total correction for TF (tetralogy of Fallot) at 3 years of age. At 8 years of age she underwent reoperation because of severe PR (pulmonary regurgitation) and RVOT (right ventricular outflow tract) aneurysm. This time she received a homograft. A year later because of RVOT aneurysm and homograft degeneration causing PR and heart failure she had a xenograft implanted, but the RVOT was not repaired. These frames are after the second operation.

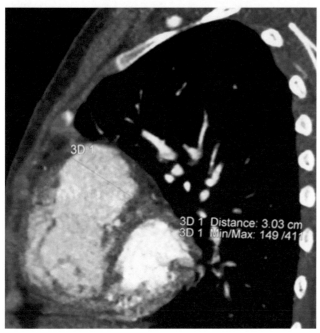

Figure 192: Note gross dilation of the RVOT due to RVOT patch aneurysm, causing RV failure.

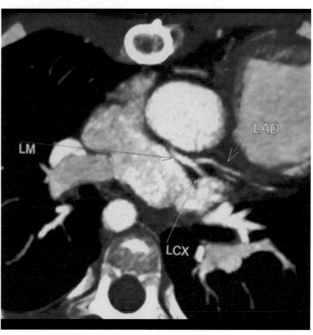

Figure 194: In all cases of TF going for total correction, coronary arteries must be studied.

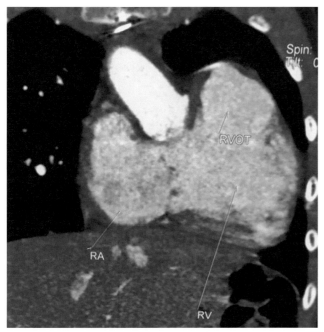

Figure 193: Note RA(right atrial),RV(right ventricular), and RVOT enlargement due to PR (pulmonary regurgitation) and RVOT aneurysm.

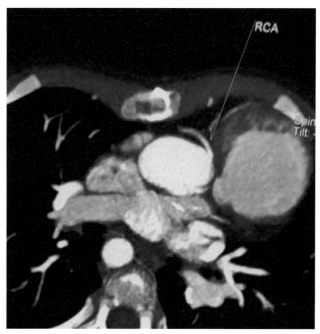

Figure 195: In all cases of TF going for total correction, coronary arteries must be studied.

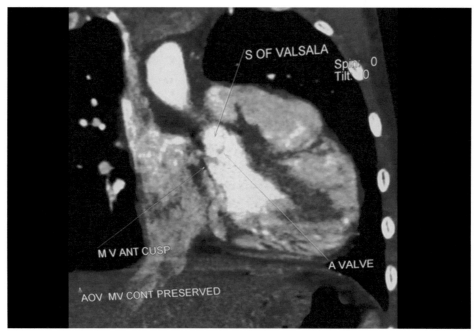

Figure 196: In all cases of tetralogy of Fallot, one must look at aorto-mitral valve continuity, thus ruling out double outlet right ventricle.

Case study: MH #089

Patient is a 37-year-old male followed since age 29 years of age. He had right hemiplegia following his first operation for correction of the tetralogy of Fallot as a child.

The patient had a porcine xenograft implanted at 29 years of age because of severe PR (pulmonary regurgitation) and RV (right ventricular) failure. This study shows the degenerated xenograft with gross enlargement of the MPA (main pulmonary artery) and main branches. RVOT (right ventricular outflow tract) is dilated and the strut of the degenerated xenograft are shown below. After this study at age 34 he had a metallic valve implanted and RVOT aneurysm was repaired.

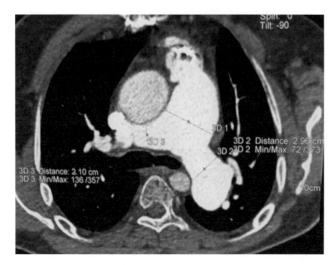

Figure 197: Dilated MPA and branches: MPA 2.96, RPA 2.10 and LPA 2.96 cm in diameter respectively.

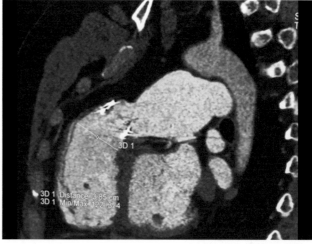

Figure 198: Aneurysmally dilated RVOT 3.85 cm in diameter. Strut of the degenerated porcine valve and dilated MPA.

Case study :ZH #092

Patient is a 17-year-old girl followed since15 months of age. She had a history of Kawasaki disease at 12 months of age. Her physical exam and chest X-ray were unremarkable, however EKG showed negative T-waves in aVF. A large aneurysm was noted by echocardiography in the LCA.

At 8 and 14 years of age she had CT angio study.

The following frames show her coronary artery pathology at 14 yrs of age.

LM (left main coronary artery) stem was within normal limits.

LAD (left anterior descending coronary artery)showed aneurysm in the mid-portion with thrombosis, but it was patent distally.

LCX (left circumflex coronary artery) was patent with proximal aneurysm.

RCA(right coronary artery) was dominant with aneurysm in the proximal and mid-portions.The distal part of the RCA was fed by collaterals.

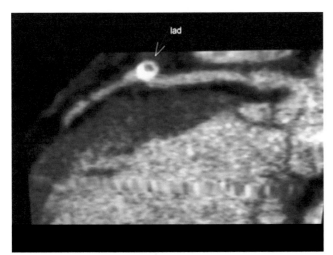

Figure 199: LAD aneurysm in the mid-portion with thrombosis, but patent distally.

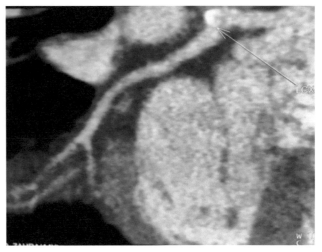

Figure 200: LCX, patent with proximal aneurysm.

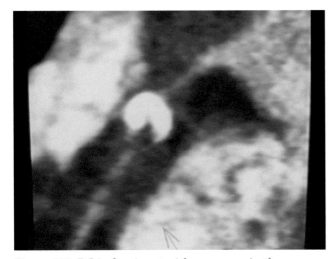

Figure 201: RCA, dominant with aneurysm in the proximal and mid-portion.

Case Study:ZA #093

Patient is a 33 -year-old female first seen at 4 years of age.She had situs solitus, mesocardia, tricuspid atresia type IIC, juxtaposed atrial appendages, d-TGV, severe pulmonary and sub-pulmonary stenosis. Preoperative PA (pulmonary arterial) pressure was 14/11 mmHg with a mean of 13 mmHg. At the age of 10 years she underwent Fontan operation ie TCPC (total cavopulmonary anastomosis), a fenestrated lateral Goretex tunnel and enlargement of the ASD (atrial septal defect). She was lost to follow-up until 25 years of age when she came with her husband, asking regarding advisability of pregnancy.

Being blue,O2 saturation 71%, with EF(ejection fraction by simpson's method) of 51% she was advised against pregnancy, however not following the advice, she became pregnant three times and aborted each time. This CT angio study was performed at 27 years of age.

CT angios are remarkable by rapid filling of the LA(left atrium) from dye injection into the right arm vein pointing to large right-to-left shunt via fenestrum.

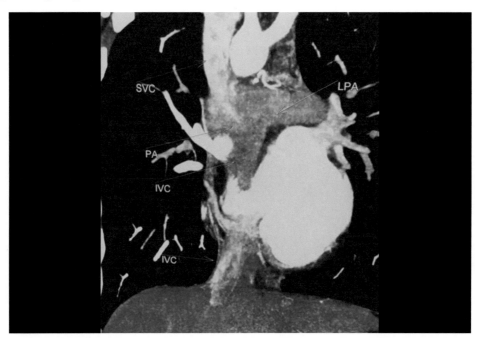

Figure 202: Situs solitus, mesocardia. IVC empties into the RPA via a lateral
fenestrated tunnel. SVC is anastomosed to the RPA. Note rapid filling of
the LA due to massive R-L shunting via fenestrum and enlarged IVC, a
sign of poor result.

Case Study: MMK #094

Patient is a 38-day-old boy who was seen for cynosis and heart failure. He had severe RVH(right ventricular hypertrophy) on EKG and cor bovinum on chest X-ray.TAPVD (total anomalous venous drainage) was diagnosed by echocardiography with a TR (tricuspid regurgitation) of 53 mmHg. CT angio showed TAPVD into the CS(coronary sinus).

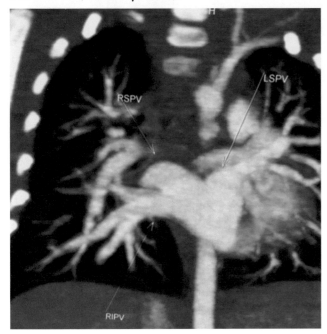

Figure 203: TAPVD into CS.

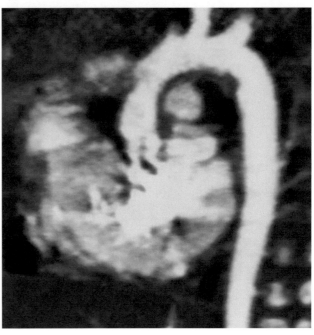

Figure 205: Normal LV and aorta. No PDA,no CoA.

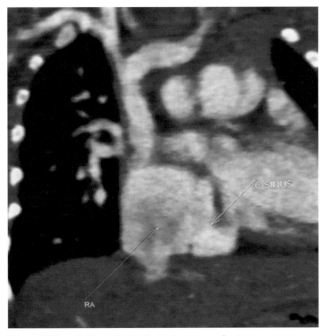

Figure 204: Enlarged CS draining into the RA.

Case Study:MMZ #097

Patient is a 3-month-old boy with cyanosis and frequent blue spells. His physical exam, EKG chest-X ray and echocardiography showed tetralogy of Fallot (TF). CT angio performed prior to a shunt. At 18 months of age he underwent total correction. Presently he is 3 1/2 years of age,fully active with good cardiac repair.

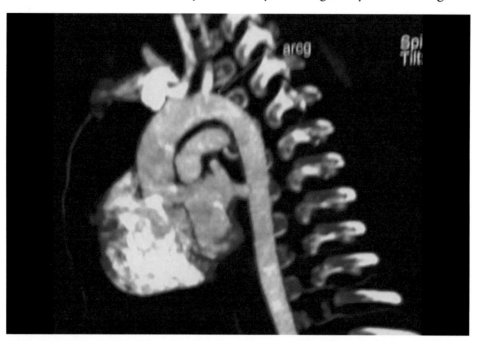

Figure 206: TF, with hypertrophied RV (right ventricle) and dextroposed aortic root and VSD (ventricular septal defect).

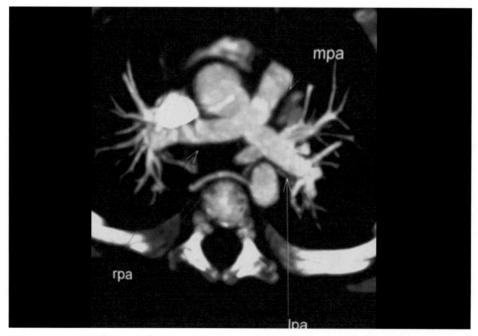

Figure 207: MPA (main pulmonary artery) and main branches of adequate size.

Case study:HM #098

Patient is a 15-month-old girl with diagnosis of large membranous VSD (ventricular septal defect) followed since 31 days of age. This study was performed prior to total correction of the VSD.

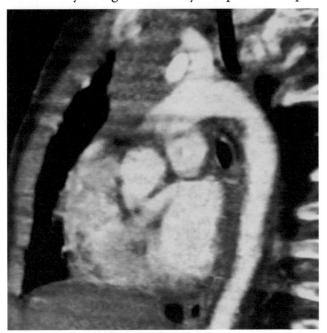 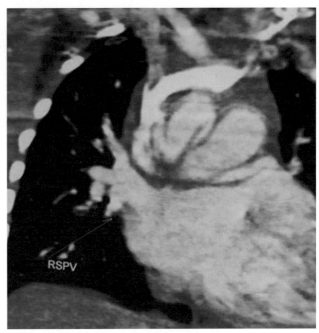

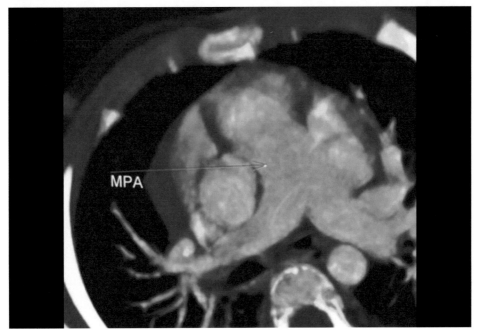

Figure 208: Note biventricular enlargement, normal aorta, normal pulmonary venous return, and engorged but normal pulmonary arteries.

Case study:PA #100

Patient is a 5 1/2-year-old boy followed since 8 months of age with a diagnosis of a large membranous VSD(ventricular septal defect) with moderate shunt. He has bicuspid aortic valve but there is neither aortic stenosis(AS) nor aortic regurgitation (AR). At 2 years of age he showed mild AR but no AS. Over the years the VSD became smaller with a septal aneurysm, and the shunt is small now with a QP/QS= 1.2/1 by echo-Doppler method. He has also developed a subaortic web but with no AS. He was operated and subaortic web was resected and VSD was closed. Because of an iatrogenic aorto-RVOT fistula, he was reoperated and the fistula was closed a week after the first operation

The following frame is from the study before the first operation.At present he has moderate AR with 17 mmHg peak gradient (flow gradient) across the aortic valve. He will eventually need AVR (aortic valve replacement) at the proper time.

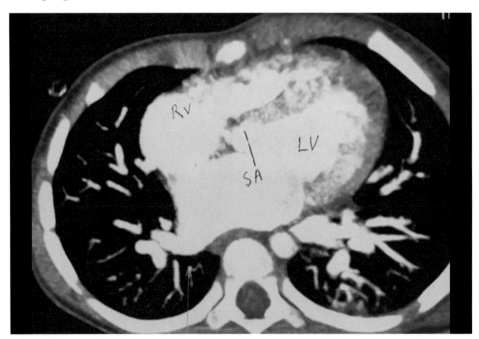

Figure 209: Note septal aneurysm (SA) making the VSD small.

Case study: MK #101

Patient is a 26-year-old male followed since 6 1/2 years of age with tetralogy of Fallot. He underwent total correction a month after the first admission. He did well but over the years till 10 years of age. After that he failed to show up for follow-up exams. Fifteen years later he showed up at 25 years of age with severe PR (pulmonary regurgitation),and grossly dilated RVOT(right ventricular outflow tract) patch causing RV (right ventricular) dysfunction.He is obese (95 Kg), not physically active, and denying symptoms. His NT-proBNP is elevated (213 pg/ml).A submaximal voluntary exercise test was grossly abnormal, due to RV (right ventricular) dsysfunction. A CT angio was performed prior to operation.

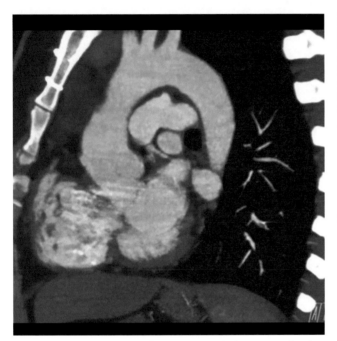

Figure 210: Lateral view showing grossly hypertrophied and dilated RV.

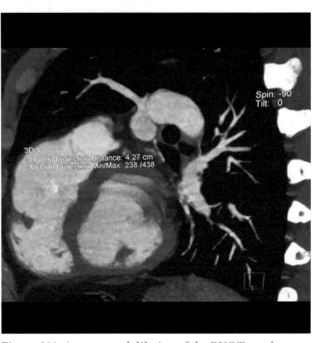

Figure 211: Aneurysmal dilation of the RVOT patch.

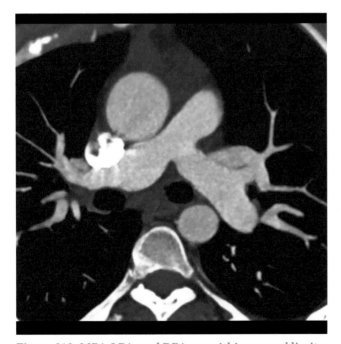

Figure 212: MPA,LPA, and RPA are within normal limits.

Case study: FY #106

Patient was a 22-year-old girl first seen at 18 months of age. She had situs inversus totalis (dextrocardia),VSD (ventricular septal defect) with pulmonary atresia, L-loop great arteries, TGV (transposition of the great vessels) and two shunts done at 6 and 10 years of age. On catheterization at 12 years of age,she had azygos continuation of IVC on the left side, huge membranous VSD, and an apical VSD, and a moderate-sized ASD (atrial septal defect).The left shunt performed at 10 years of age was patent, but the right shunt,performed at 6 years of age was clotted.LPA (left pulmonary artery) was 1.38 cm in diameter. RPA (right pulmonary artery) had origin stenosis 0.90 -1.07 cm in diameter. At 14 years of age she underwent "Rastelli" procedure elsewhere. ASD and VSD were closed, and a homograft was implanted connecting right sided LV (left ventricle) to the MPA (main pulmonary artery). She did fairly well until 22 years of age when she developed "pneumonia" for which she was treated elsewhere, but when she was seen following "therapy" she had signs and symptoms of frank heart failure and gross anemia. LV EF (left ventricular ejection fraction) was 33% and homograft showed signs of stenosis **with (infected) clots.** An emergency CT angio was performed and emergency operation to change the homograft was recommended at high risk.The surgeon refused to operate and opted for antibiotic therapy. The patient expired a few days later with final diagnosis of the **right heart bacterial endocarditis** involving the homograft.

The following frames were obtained a week before death.

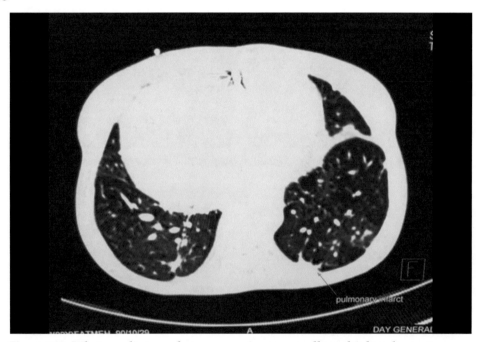

Figure 213: What was diagnosed as pneumonia was actually multiple pulmonary infarcts, from infected shower emboli from the homograft.

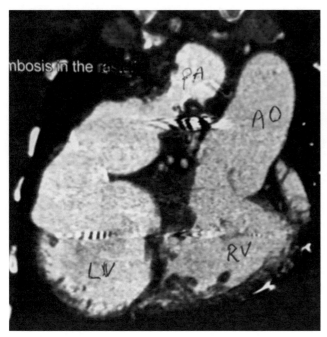

Figure 214: Figure 213: Post-op,VSD closure, and homograft connecting anatomic LV to PA stump.Note thrombosis narrowing the homograft lumen.

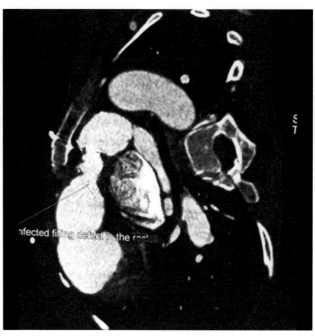

Figure 216: Infected thrombus in the homograft impinging on the lumen.

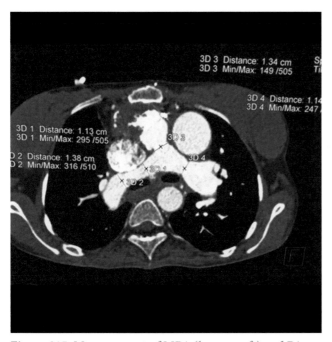

Figure 215: Measurement of MPA (homograft) and PA branches.Hypoplastic pulmonary artery system.

Case study:ZQ #105

Patient is a 14-year-old female followed since 18 months of age. She had single left ventricle,d-loop great vessels (d-TGV), severe pulmonary and subpulmonary stenosis, and juxtaposed atrial appendages. She had a left shunt at 6 years of age and a right central shunt at 10 years of age.The patient was erratic in follow-up visits and this final CT angio study was performed at 14 years of age because of increasing cyanosis and effort-intolerance. Based on this study a hybrid Fontan,ie leaving RPA (right pulmonary artery) and right central shunt alone, and ligating RPA, and a fenestrated tunnel from IVC (inferior vena cava) to the LPA (left pulmonary artery) was considered a posssible option to relieve her hypoxia. However she was lost to follow-up.

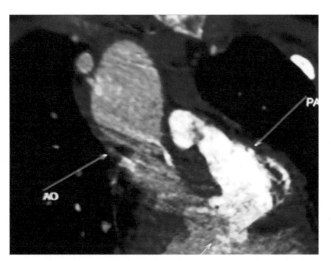

Figure 217: Figure 216:Situs solitus viscera and atria, single left ventricle (bottom arrow), d-loop great vessels, d-TGV, with severe pulmonary valvar and subpulmonary stenosis.

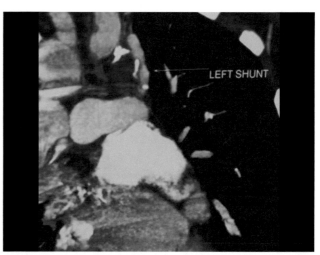

Figure 218: Small patent left shunt above LPA (left pulmonary artery).

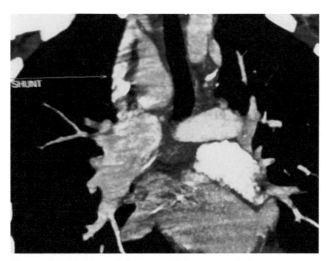

Figure 219: Patent right central shunt, top left.

Case study :MS # 103:

Patient is a 6-year-old boy with diagnosis of sinus venosus ASD (atrial septal defect). CT angio was performed which showed that patient also has partial anomalous pulmonary venous drainage (PAPVD).

Undiagnosed PAPVD could be a very unpleasant surprise at the time of total correction. CT angio is a powerful tool to prevent such an incident.

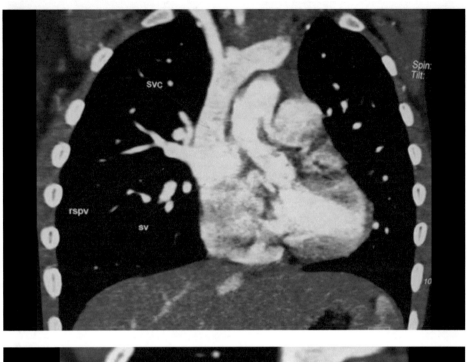

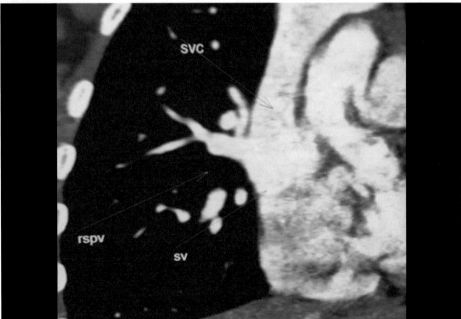

Figure 220: Note right superior pulmonary vein draining into sinus venosus just below the ostium of the superior vena cava.

Case study : KM #104

Patient is an 8-month-old baby girl who was referred with diagnosis of infantile hypercalcemia (William's syndrome). The patient had an enlarged heart on chest X-ray .Echocardiography showed supravalvar aortic stenosis with a peak gradient of 96 mmHg and small LPA (left pulmonary artery), RPA(right pulmonary artery), and peripheral pulmonary stenosis of 30 mmHg.

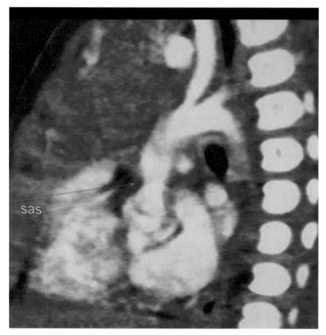

Figure 221: Supravalvar aortic stenosis.

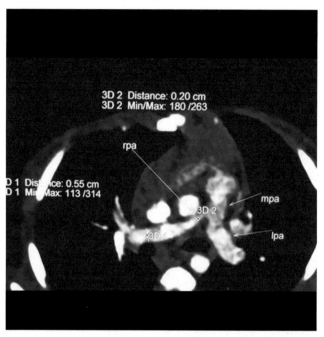

Figure 222: Small PA system and RPA origin stenosis 0.20 cm .

Case study:EK #216

Patient an asymptomatic 50-day-old female with a small PDA(patent ductus arteriosus) .

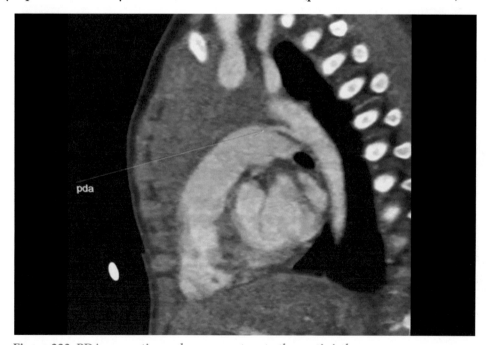

Figure 223: PDA connecting pulmonary artery to the aortic isthmus.

Case study:MA #123

Patient is a 50-day-old girl referred for a heart murmur and failure to thrive. She had murmur of mitral regurgitation, with enlarged heart on chest X-ray and LVH (left ventricular hypertrophy) with strain on EKG.Echocardiography showed massive mitral regurgitation,LVH and enlarged LA(left atrium). Her NT-proBNP was 20755 pg/ml. This patient had familial CMP(cardiomyopathy) with her mother's EKG showing negative T waves in aVF and another brother 11 years of age with gross LVH on EKG.

Although the diagnosis of CMP with massive MR of familial nature was established, a CT angio was performed to study the coronary arteries. It is a must in all cases of pediatric mitral regurgitation to rule out abnormalities of the coronaries, esp LAD (left anterior descending) arising from MPA(main pulmonary artery).In the following frames note massive LVH and normal coronary origin.

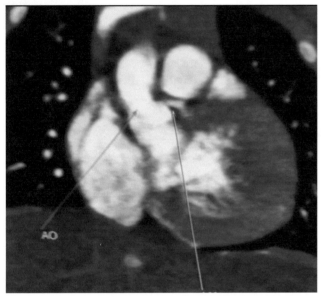

Figure 224: Normal left main coronary artery.
Note gross LVH.

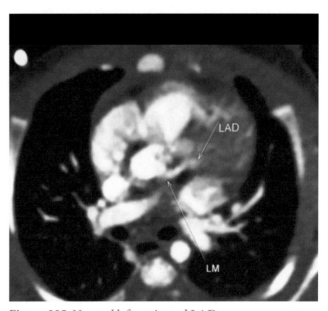

Figure 225: Normal left main and LAD

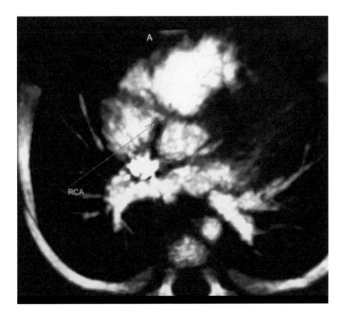

Figure 226: Normal RCA.

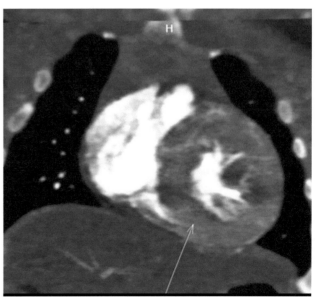

Figure 227: Note gross LVH due to HCMP.

133

Case study:YF #122

Patient is a 7-year-old boy first seen at the age of 4 1/2 years. He was operated elsewhere, for coarctation of the aorta at the age of 1 year. A diagnosis of recoarctation was made prior to the first visit and the patient was started on captopril.On physical exam pulses were normal in amplitude. Blood pressure was 90/60 mmHg in the right arm, in reclining position. On echocardiography a gradient of 40 mmHg was discovered by Doppler,proximal to the coarctation site at left subclavian artery origin. Patient had a bicuspid aortic valve with no aortic stenosis.

A CT angio was performed with the diagnosis of **pseudocoarctation** of the aorta.

CT angio is a powerful method to rule out or in recoarctation of the aorta. The incongruous diameters shown below, togther with normal pulses and blood pressure, allow ruling out recoarctation and obviating the need for catheterization.

Also see the report by Baumgartner et al, in the section of References.

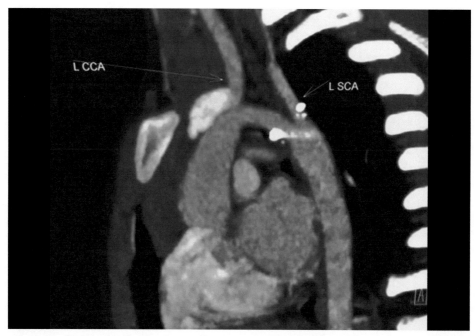

Figure 228: Note the area of apparent "recoarctation" close to the left subclavian artery. Ascending aorta is dilated as in most cases with bicuspid aortic valve.

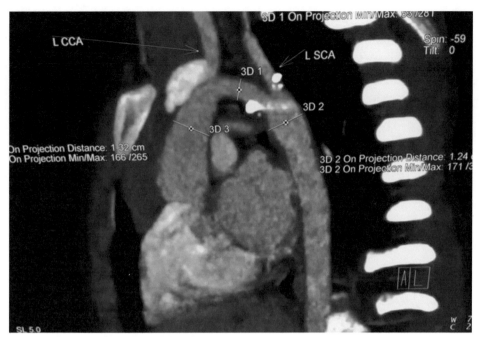

Figure 229: Ascending aorta 1.32 cm, aortic arch before isthmus 0.69 cm, aortic isthmus distal to the coarctation operation site 1.24 cm in diameter.

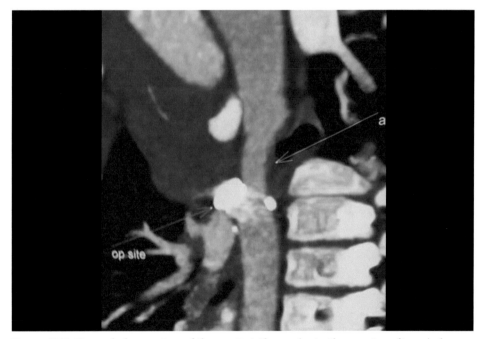

Figure 230: Curved planar view of the aortic isthmus (as in the previous figure) shows different diameters of the aorta proximal and distal to the operative site. The different shape and diameter of various segments of arteries could produce turbulence and pseudo-gradients by Doppler.

Case study: AM #120

Patient is a 6-year-old female followed since 1 month of age. She had situs solitus, single ventricle,d-TGV (transposition of the great vessels) with increased pulmonary blood flow and heart failure. Pulmonary artery banding (PAB) and BH(Blalock-Hanlon) operations were performed at 40 days of age.

At 26 months of age PA band was very tight, there was no LSVC(left superior vena cava) and O2 saturation was 80% by pulse oximetry in room air.

A PA band peak gradient of 76 mmHg and systemic systolic pressure of 95/60 mmHg, predicted a peak systolic PA (pulmonary artery) pressure of 20 mmHg. Echo-derived PAWP (pulmonary artery wedge pressure) was 15 mmHg.

A two-stage Fontan operation was proposed and patient underwent a right Glenn shunt.A year later a CT angio was performed in preparation for lateral fenesrated tunnel,ie the 2nd stage of Fontan operation. CT angio frames prior to 2nd stage of Fontan operation:

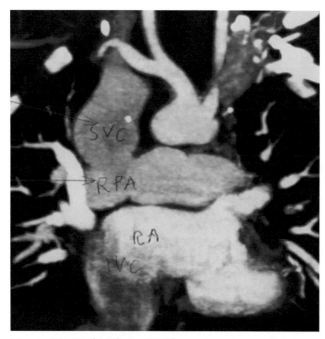

Figure 231: Right Glenn: SVC(superior vena cava) anastomosed to the RPA(right pulmonary artery).

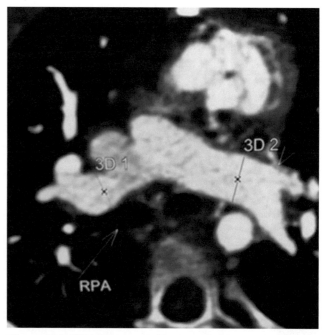

Figure 232: RPA 1.02 cm in diameter, LPA 1.28 cm in diameter.

A 20 mm Dacron tunnel with a fenestrum, 5 mm in diameter was performed at 3 years of age.

Patient is now in good shape and is fully active. Her ejection fraction is suboptimal (54% Simpson's rule), and she has 88-90% O2 saturation. There is therefore a moderate RL shunt at the fenestral level. She is on digitalis and sildenafil.

Case study: NA #120

Patient is a 27-year-old female first seen at 8 1/2 years of age, followed elsewhere since 1 year of age. During the first visit she was diagnosed to have bicuspid aortic valve, severe aortic stenosis rule out coarctation of the aorta. Aortic valve peak gradient by Doppler was ≥ 100 mmHg. She was catheterized and was found to have LV pressure of 210 mmHg and aortic systolic pressure of 120 mmHg. There was aortic arch kinking with 10 mmHg peak gradient on pull-back. Operation was recommended and aortic valvotomy was performed . Eight months postoperatively she was seen again with AS (aortic stenosis) peak gradient by Doppler ≥ 67 mmHg. There was minimal AR as well. At ten years of age the result of operation was poor with severe aortic stenosis PG ≥ 101 mmHg by Doppler. Repeat catheterization and operation were advised, however the patient disappeared. Seventeen years later she showed up again,with her husband. She was now a sports club instructor denying symptoms!! She had low pulse pressure in all four extremities. Her EKG showed LVH(left ventricular hypertrophy) with strain in the inferior leads. She had all the clinical signs of severe aortic valvar stenosis. Aortic peak gradient was ≥ 90 mmHg.Her echoderived PAWP was ≥15 mmHg.

The following CT angio was performed prior to operation. The study was performed but patient did not show up, as of this date 2 years.

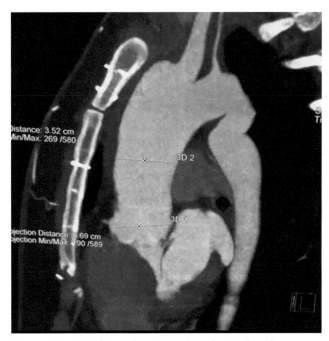

Figure 233: Thick dysplastic aortic valve. Dilated ascending aorta 3.52 cm.Aortic isthmus kinking.

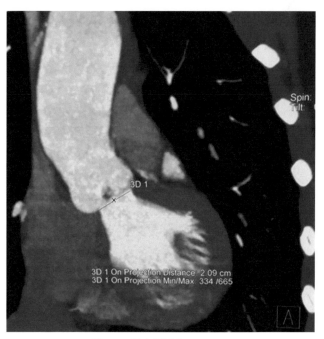

Figure 234: Thick dysplastic aortic valve, with gross LV hypertrophy.

Case Study:MRMQ #131

Patient is a 17-year-old male followed since 22 months of age with the diagnosis of Taussig-Bing anomaly ie DORV(double outlet right ventricle) with d-TGV(transposition of the great vessels), PS (pulmonary stenosis) and severe MR (mitral regurgitation) due to MV(mitral valve) cleft.His VSD(ventricular septal defect) was closed and a Rastelli procedure was performed using a homograft elsewhere, but the mitral valve was not repaired.

At 7 1/2 years of age the homograft was degenerated and fully calcified,with 79 mmHg peak gradient by Doppler. His RV(right ventricular) pressure was 90/0-8 mmHg during catheterization. A repeat operation was advised, to close a residual VSD, repair mitral valve and replace the homograft.

Following operation at 7 and 7/12 years of age,homograft PG(peak gradient) was 31 mmHg, MV showed mild to moderate MR. Her NT-proBNP 322 pg/ml. The patient was followed with anticongestive heart failure medications.

At 11 year of age homograft was degenerated and mitral regurgitation persisted. A third operation was advised.This time a valved conduit # 23 porcine was implanted and MV was repaired again. There was no PS/PR postop and MR was mild. Heart failure improved postoperatively.

At 14 yrs of age patient was obese (66 Kg), MR was mild but TR (tricuspid regurgitation) was noted. A CT angio was performed. RVOT (right ventricular outflow tract) was wnl (1.99 cm in diameter). The conduit was calcified. The valve peak gradient was 60 mmHg by Doppler. The patch on the LVOT (left ventricular outflow tract), between LA(left atrium),RA(right atrium) and aortic root was aneurysmal, measuring 1.94x2.03 cm.

LMCA(left main coronary artery) and RCA(right coronary artery) arose from the sinus of Valsalva above the non-coronary cusp of the aortic valve.

This time a metallic valve was implanted. Presently at 17 years of age. He is obese (76 Kg). There is no heart failure and the valve is functioning well.

CT angio frames before the last operation are shown below:

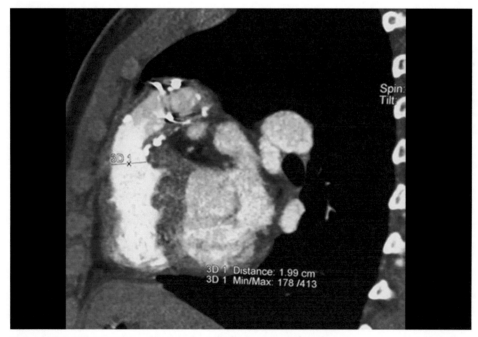

Figure 235: RVOT 1.99 wnl, severely calcified xenograft valve.

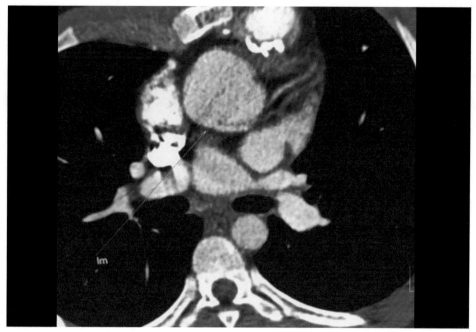

Figure 236: LMCA and RCA arising from the noncoronary cusp of the sinus of Valsalva.

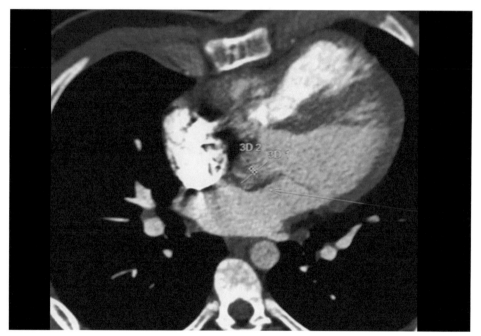

Figure 237: LVOT patch aneurysm between RA,LA and AO measuring 1.94x2.03 cm.

Case Study:HP # 132

Pt is a 3 1/2-year-old girl followed since 2 months of age with a small VSD (ventricular septal defect),stretched PFO (patent foramen ovale), valvar PS (pulmonary stenosis), dysplastic pulmonic valve and aneurysmal dilation of the MPA (main pulmonary artery).

At one year of age she had a stretched PFO,and 50 mmHg peak gradient across the membranous VSD. She had 55 mmHg peak gradient across an anomalous RV (right ventricular) band and 35 mmHg peak gradient across the dysplastic stenotic pulmonic valve. The patient was operated at 19 months of age. At operation the PFO was closed. The VSD was closed.The stenotic anomalous RV band was resected. MPA was aneurysmally dilated,however it was left untouched. The pulmonic valve though dysplastic was mildly stenotic and therefore it was not touched. Postoperatively the pulmonic stenosis PG (peak gradient) was 26 mmHg and trivial PR(pulmonary regurgitation) was present.

At 3 1/2 yr of age the patient is fully active and asymptomatic,with mild PR (pulmonary regurgitation) (15 mmHg), mild pulmonary stenosis PS (17 mmHg peak gradient) and aneurysmally dilated MPA.

CT angio frames preop:

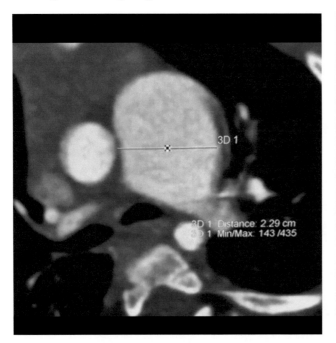 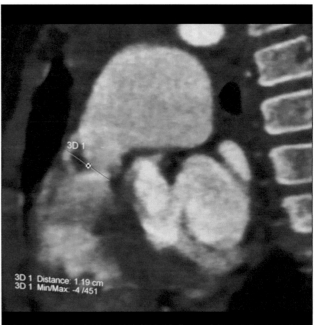

Figure 238: Dysplastic pulmonic valve with aneurysmal dilation of the MPA.

Case study: SJ #146

Patient a male adolescent was first seen at 19 years of age. The father stated that a diagnosis of coarctation of the aorta was made at 9 years of age. A balloon dilation was performed. Neither pre-, nor post-procedure data could be secured. Patient's chief complaint was pain in the right leg when walking fast. Blood pressure including a 24-hour blood pressure monitoring were within normal limits. Right femoral, posterior tibialis and dorsalis pedis pulses were impalpable. The physical examination was otherwise unremarkable. EKG was within normal limits. Echocardiography was also unremarkable, including Doppler examination of the ascending and descending aorta. PA (pulmonary artery) flow was 7 mmHg with no PR (pulmonary regurgitation). AAo(ascending aortic) flow was 12 mmHg and descending aortic flow was 19 mmHg.

This case represents a major complication of the interventional technique, with stripping of the iliac artery intima and subsequent obliteration of flow.

A CT angio was performed:

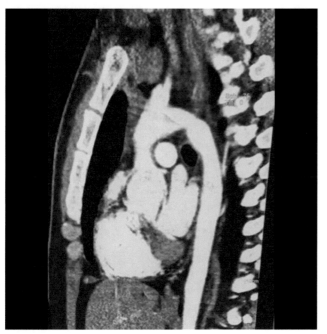

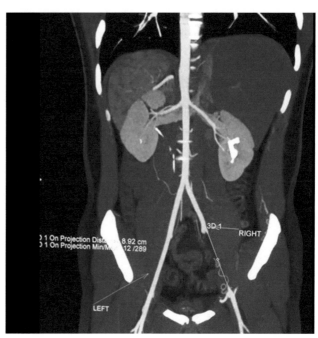

Figure 239: Normal aortic arch and isthmus. Proximal aortic isthmus 1.67 cm, and distal aortic isthmus 1.41 cm in diameter.

Figure 240: Right iliac artery cut-off, fed by collaterals.

Case study:MMQ #157

Patient is a 6-year-old boy first seen at 3 years of age. He had a brother with Ebstein's disease and cardiomyopathy who died suddenly.Another brother had ASD(atrial septal defect) which was operated. The patient was asymptomatic but had signs of Pierre-Robin syndrome plus mental and motor retardation. Physical examination, chest X-ray, EKG and echocardiography established the diagnosis of a large ASD secundum. RV(right ventricle) (2.8 cm end-diastolic diameter), RA(right atrium) (21 ml), and PA (pulmonary artery) were enlarged. The medial cusp of the tricuspid valve was very small on echocardiography however its attachment site was normal.There was no tricuspid regurgitation. Tissue-Doppler examination showed posterior left ventricular wall, RV (right ventricular) and ventricular septal myocardial dysfunction. His ASD was closed surgically shortly after the first visit.

CT angio showed a large ASD secundum type,with normal pulmonary venous drainage. The tricuspid valve was normal as shown on the following frames.

Presently he is asymptomatic, fully active. However he has developed sinoatraial block or sinus arrest on EKG and Holter examination. He is being followed for subclinical CMP(cardiomyopathy) and sinoatrial block.

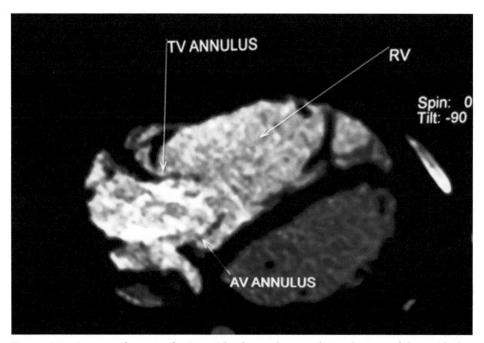

Figure 241: Apparently normal tricuspid valve and normal attachment of the medial and lateral cusps.

Case study :MA #158

Patient is a 22-year old female followed since 3 months of age. She had valvar PS (pulmonic stenosis) initially with 59 mmHg peak gradient and a small membranous VSD (ventricular septal defect). At 3 1/2 year of age she was catheterized and operated elsewhere. She showed up one year later at 4 1/2 year of age. Echocardiography showed no VSD, no PS and no PR (pulmonary regurgitation). Again she was lost to follow-up, and showed up at 11 years of age. She had CRBBB on EKG, and on echocardiography she had mild PR but no PS. Lost to follow-up again and showed up at 21 years of age with chief complaint of DOE (dyspnea on exertion) and palpitation.On physical exam she had wide fixed split S2, 2/6 diastolic murmur of PR(pulmonary regurgitation). Echocardiography showed moderate PR (14 mmHg), dilated RVOT(right ventricular outflow tract) 2.9 cm, plus moderate to severe TR (tricuspid regurgitation). RA(right atrial) volume was 32 ml/m², RVEF (right ventricular ejection fraction) was 56% (Simpson's rule). Her NT-proBNP was elevated she was treated medically.

A CT angio confirmed the clinical findings and she is up for pulmonary valve replacement and TV (tricuspid valve) repair or replacement. Due to the divorce of parents the operation is postponded till the date of this report.

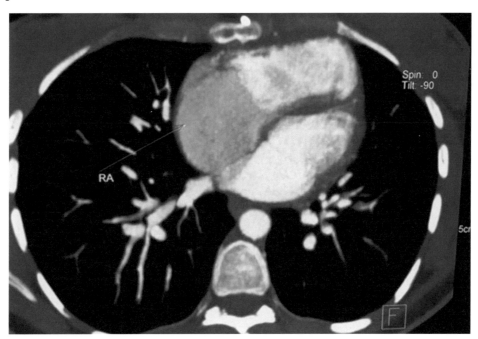

Figure 242: Dilated RA.

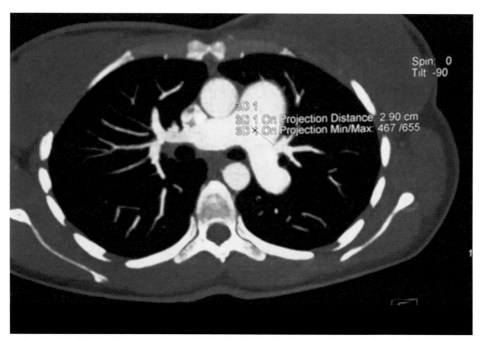

Figure 243: Dilated MPA.

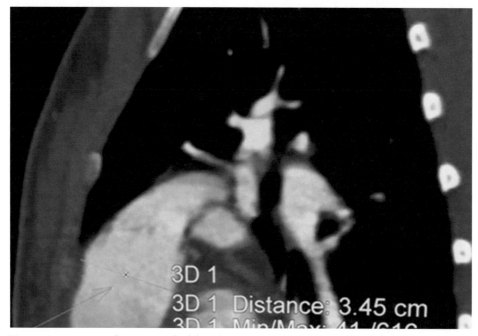

Figure 244: Arrow shows grossly dilated RVOT, 3.45 cm in diameter.

Case Study: TA #160

This case serves as a prototype of the majority of our patients with tetrtalogy of Fallot who have undergone total correction with RVOT(right ventricular outflow tract) patch or transannular patch in infancy or childhood. If the patch is too generous (initially with remarkably good results), several years later the patients go in right heart failure due to RVOT patch aneurysm, and severe PR(pulmonary regurgitation), eventually leading to RV(right ventricular) failure with secondary massive TR (tricuspid regurgitation). Therefore the patch must be carefully measured at the time of total correction.

This patient is a 22-year-old girl who is architect student and unmarried. She has been followed since 6 months of age.She had a left Goretex shunt at 9 months of age. At 3 years of age she underwent total correction. At 4 years of age she had moderate PR.

At 9 years of age RVOT was dilated, measuring 3.4 cm in diameter.Moderate TR was noted at 10 years of age. The patient was catheterized at 11 years of age.She had free PR, so that injection of contrast material in the RPA (right pulmonary artery) opacified MPA (main pulmonary artery) and the RV(right ventricle). RV pressure was 50/0-2,and PA (pulmonary artery) pressure was 35/0-2 mmHg. She was operated at 11 years of age with a #21 porcine valve replacing the pulmonic valve. One year later the xenograft valve peak gradient was 45 mmHg by Doppler. The patient was catheterized at 13 years of age. This study showed and an RV pressure of 90/0-15 mmHg,and PA pressure of 25-30 mmHg, (mean 25)15 mmHg. The xenograft was replaced at 14 years of age with another one. The peak gradient across the pulmonic valve was 24 mmHg by Doppler postoperatively. She had frequent attacks of SVT(supraventricular tachycardia), which responded to treatment with beta-blocker.At 15 years of age she had moderate PR with peak gradient of 22 mmHg.Also there was moderate TR with 47 mmHg peak gradient by Doppler.

At 17 years of age she had 29 mmHg peak gradient across the pulmonic valve with RVOT measuring 2.6 cm in diameter, moderate PR and TR.

At 19 years of age peak gradient across the valve was 46 mmHg. RVOT measured 3.6 cm in diameter, RV EF (right ventricular ejection fraction) was 37% by Simpson's rule. There was moderate TR with PG gradient of 37 mmHg, RA volume index of 47 ml/m^2, and NT-proBNP 300 pg/ml. She complained of SOB (shortness of breath) and DOE (dyspnea on exertion). An exercise test (voluntary, submaximal 85%, Bruce protocol) showed subnormal response.

At the of 19 years of age, in preparation for another operation, the patient quite understadably very apprehensive, underwent a CT angio study, the results of which supported the clinical findings.

Following this study at 20 years of age, she underwent reoperation. This time, a St-Jude's metallic was implanted for the degenerated porcine valve, and RVOT was repaired. Two years postop she is doing fine. She is asysmptomatic. PG across the valve is 11 mmHg by Doppler.

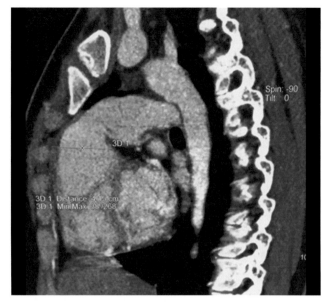

Figure 245: RVOT aneurysmal 4.15 cm in diameter.

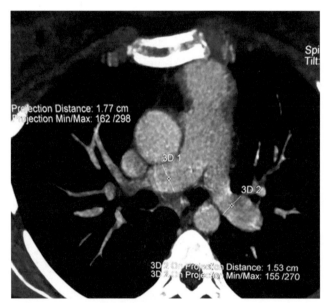

Figure 246: Normal aorta, dilated MPA.

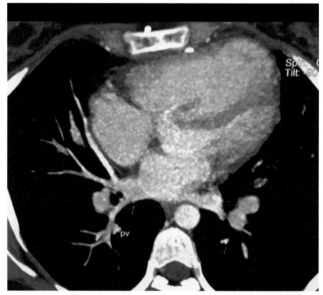

Figure 247: Enlarged RA and RV, normal pulmonary venous return.

[**Corollary:** 1-The **homografts** prepared locally in **developing countries**, should not be trusted, because of possible **poor treatment** of the harvested specimens and **lax execution** of the preparation protocol. (**Technician's failure.)**

2- **Xenograft failures,** as noted in this case, are due to **surgeon's poor treatment of the valve during operation**. The comments by Carpentier, very astutely and delicately expressed in his commentary on a report by Flameng et al. are quite appropriate for cases noted by the author. The entire commentary and the paper by Flameng et al deserve to be read in full, until one appreciates, the magnitude of the problem of using bioprosthesis in the young patients in developing countries. Also see the following case studies reported in this monograph, for appreciating the magnitude of the problem. MH#089,PN#087,KR#078,MRMQ#131] (JGS)

Case study: KX #235

Patient is a 9-year-old boy followed since 3 1/2 yrs of age.He was planned to have balloon pulmonary valvoplasty and was referred for evaluation. He had a wide, but not fixed split S2. His EKG was wnl (within normal limits).On echocardiography he had a dysplastic, thick pulmonic valve and a dilated MPA (main pulmonary artery). There was 19 mmHg peak gradient across the pulmonic valve. Scheduled balloon valvoplasty was advised against, and the patient was advised to have yearly check-ups. He showed up 3 years later, at the age of 6 years. His EKG was again wnl. PS (pulmonary stenosis) peak gradient was 23 mmHg and there was mild PR (pulmonary regurgitation). Again the patient did not follow advice and came back at 8 1/2 years of age. At this time he had significant PR with ectatic MPA.

A CT angio was performed..

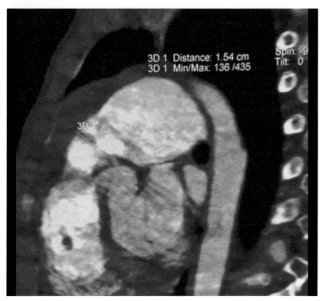

Figure 248: Dysplastic pulmonic valve, valve ring 1.54 cm in diameter.

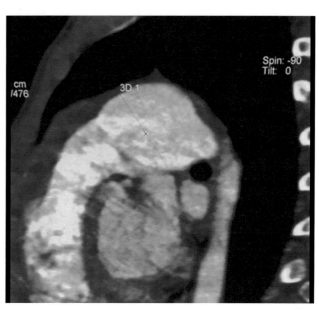

Figure 249: Ectatic MPA 3.30 cm in diameter.

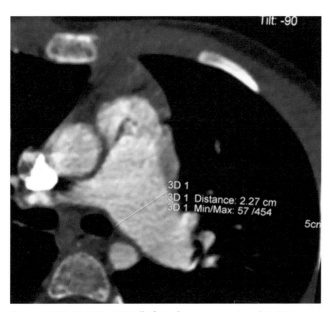

Figure 250: Ectatic LPA(left pulmonary artery) 2.27 cm in diameter.

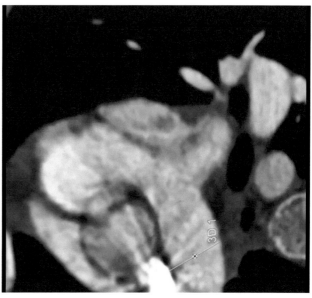

Figure 251: RPA (right pulmonary artery) diameter 1.62 cm, wnl.

Case study: PFX # 165

Patient is a 2-year-old girl followed since 8 days of age. The patient has mental and motor retardation. She had a PDA (patent ductus arteriosus) which closed around 6 months of age. She has Taussig-Bing anomaly, ie DORV,TGV(double outlet right ventricle with transposition of the great vessels).She also has severe PS (pulmonary stenosis). Because of severe hypoxia a BH (Blalock-Hanlon) operation and a shunt were advised. These frames of CT angio were obtained prior to operation at the age of 6 months.

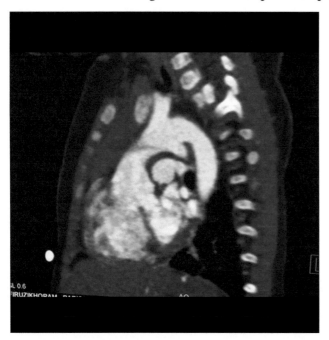
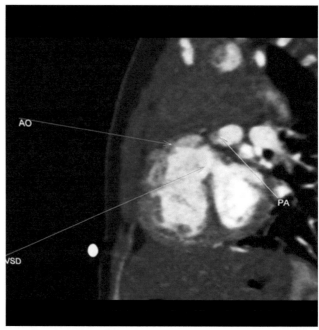

Figure 252: Note VSD,DORV with TGV,anterior aorta and posterior PA.

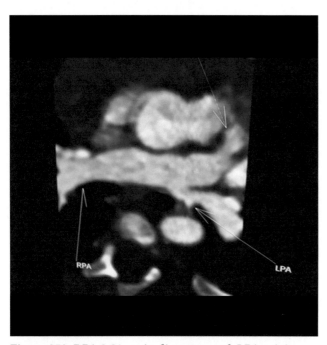

Figure 253: RPA 0.81 cm in diameter, wnl. LPA origin stenosis 0.38 cm in diameter.

Case study: AB # 164

Patient a 4-month-old boy was referred for a heart murmur. He was asymptomatic and his growth was wnl(within normal limits). Chest X-ray and EKG were wnl. A 2/6 continuous murmur was audible at midprecordium. Echocardiography showed a continuous flow in the RV (right ventricular) apex. At 14 months of age a CT angio was performed. Left main coronary artery was grossly dilated and its origin measured 0.52 cm in diameter. A tortuous LAD,with distal aneurysm emptied into the RV apex. Two coronary ostia were noted on the left side. RCA and LCX were wnl. LAD origin ligation was recommended.

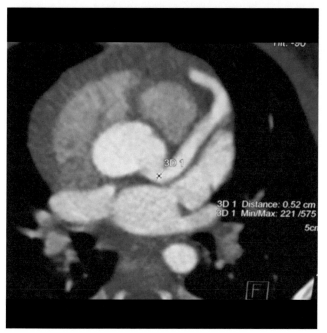

Figure 254: Left main coronary artery dilated with ostium measuring 0.52 cm in diameter.

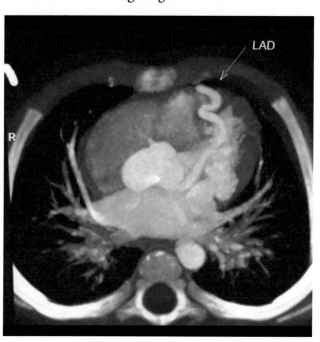

Figure 255: Tortuous LAD emptying into the RV apex.

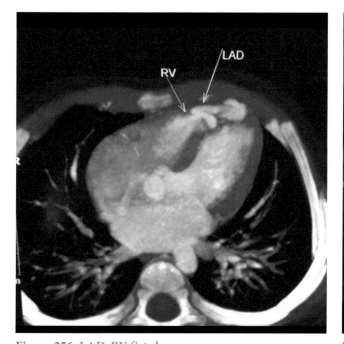

Figure 256: LAD-RV fistula.

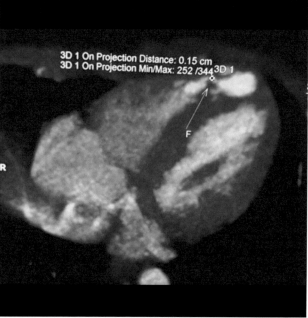

Figure 257: LAD-RV apex fistula orifice 0.15 cm in diameter.

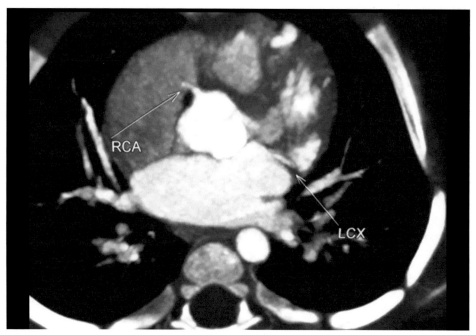

Figure 258: Normal origin of the LCX and RCA are shown in this frame.

Case study: EA # 169

Patient is a 14 month-old-girl referred for a heart murmur. Pertinent findings were failure to thrive (weight 6.5 Kg) and biventricular hypertrophy noted on EKG. A PDA (patent ductus arteriosus) was detected on echocardigraphy. A CT angio was performed, which showed a large PDA. Other incidental findings were left common carotid origin from the right brachiocephalic artery and a left SVC (superior vena cava) draining into the coronary sinus. Post-op (PDA ligation and division) the patient had an uneventful course.

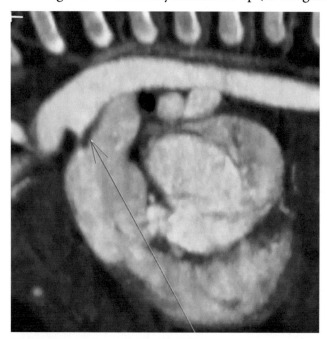

Figure 259: Arrow points to the PDA.

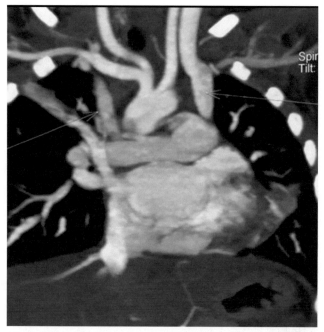

Figure 260: This frame shows left SVC and left common carotid artery originating from the right brachiocephalic artery (bovine fashion)

Case study: MST # 168

Patient is a 9-year-old boy who had recently undgone stent implantation for relief of the coarctation of the aorta(CoA). He had CVA(cerbrovascular accident) post-intervention from which he has partially recovered. His right arm systolic pressure was 140 mmHg and left arm was 80 mmHg. His femoral pulses were normal.

CT angio showed a small aortic arch (1.01 cm in diameter). A stent in the isthmus for relief of COA which is small (0.65 cm in diameter) and distal aorta measuring 1.56 cm in diameter. The origin of the left subclavian artery was impinged upon by the stent. Ascending aorta was 1.92 cm and descending aorta 1.28 cm in diameter.Thus stent caused proximal hypertension as well as disturbing the left subclavian artery flow.

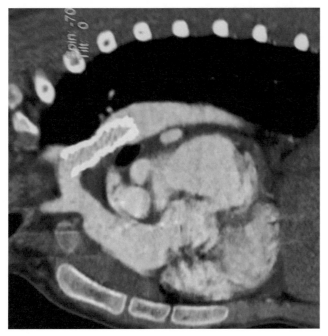

Figure 261: Stented coarctation of the aorta. See the text.

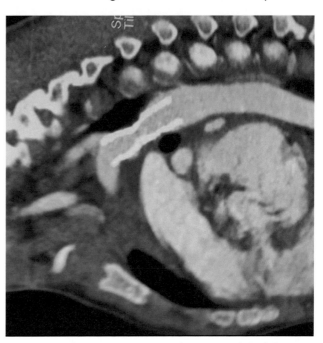

Figure 262: Stent impinging on the origin of the left subclavian artery.

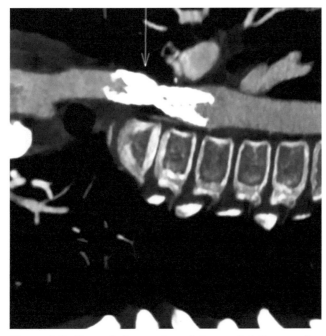

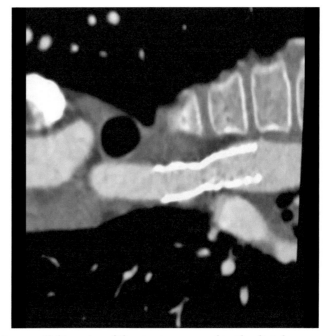

Figure 263: Curved planar view of the aortic isthmus, showing small diameter of the stent compared to the distal isthmus.

Case study: ET # 167

Patient is an asymptomatic 3-year-old male referred for a heart murmur. He has a small midseptal VSD (ventricular septal defect) and severe valvar pulmonic stenosis, with Doppler peak gradient ≥98 mmHg. A CT angio was performed. Aneurysmal LPA(left pulmonary artery) was an incidental finding.

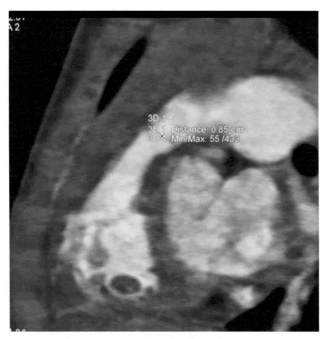

Figure 264: Severe RVH due to valvar PS.

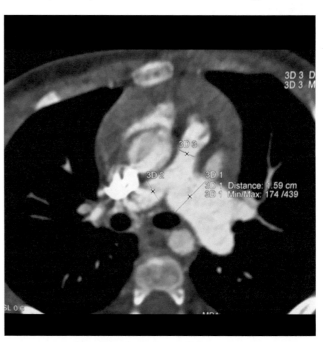

Figure 265: MPA (3D 3) measured 0.65 cm in diameter. RPA (3D 2) 0.88 cm in diameter.LPA aneurysmal 1.59 cm in diameter.

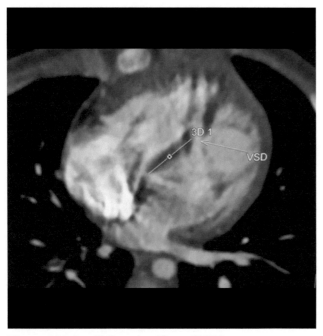

Figure 266: Small (2mm) midseptal VSD.

Case study: AH # 174

Patient is a one-month-old baby boy referred for heart failure. Truncus arteriosus type I or II was diagnosed by clinical and echocardiographic examination.

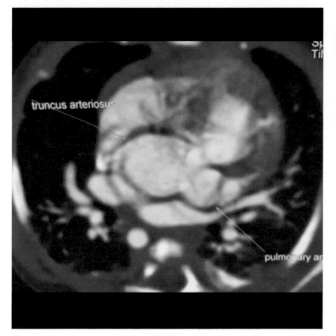

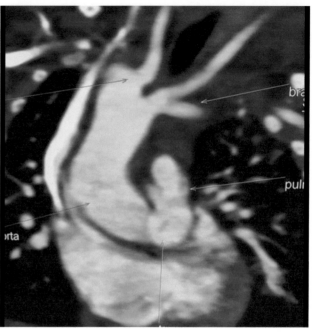

Figure 267: Truncus arteriosus type I giving rise to the pulmonary artery and the aorta. Top left arrow common carotid artery and top right arrow brachiocephalic artery.

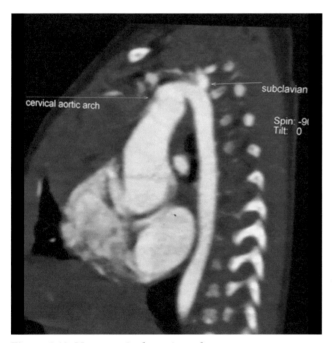

Figure 268: Note cervical aortic arch.

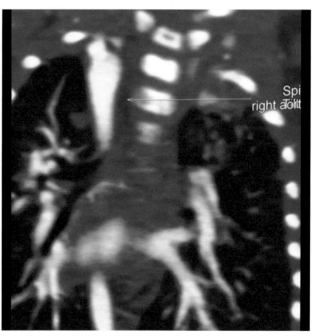

Figure 269: Note right aortic arch.

Case study: MSS # 179

Patient is a 25-year-old male,followed since 3 1/2 years of age. He had a large membranous VSD (ventricular septal defect) and severe PS(pulmonary stenosis) which was totally corrected at 4 years of age with a transannular patch.

Ever since he has been followed at outpatient department. At 19 years of age the patch was aneurysmal, RV(right ventricle) and RVOT(right ventricular outflow tract) were dilated with severe PR(pulmonary regurgitation).He was catheterized and revision operation with pulmonic valve replacement was recommended. He was lost to follow-up and showed up at 24 years of age,with SOB (shortness of breath) and DOE (dyspnea on exertion). A CT angio was performed. Following this study pulmonic valve was replaced with a metallic valve and RVOT was repaired. He is out of heart failure and active .

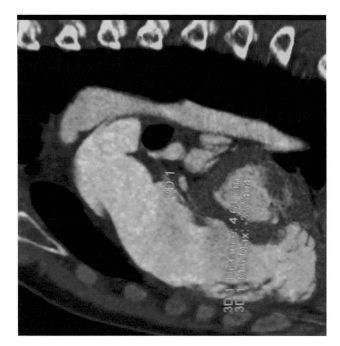 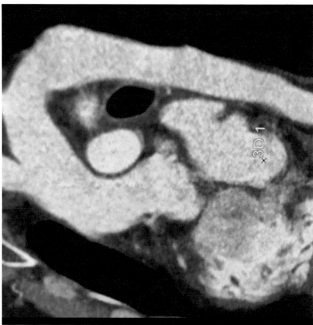

Figure 270: RVOT is aneurysmally dilated (4.61 cm in diameter),RV is hypertrophied and dilated.

Case study: SS # 187

Patient is a 17-year-old female who underwent Senning operation for d-TGV without VSD (ventricular septal defect).

Pulmonary veins and SVC-IVC baffles are shown in the following CT angio frames.

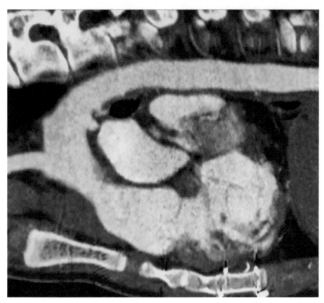

Figure 271: d-TGV with anterior aorta arising from the right ventricle and pulmonary artery posteriorly arising from the left ventricle.

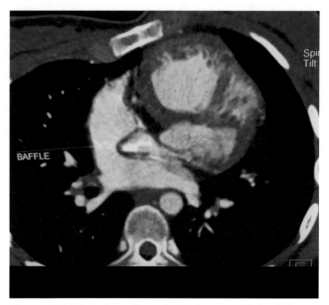

Figure 272: Fish-shaped opacity in front and left of the spine shows PV-baffle diverting pulmonary venous flow to the RV. The small triagular opacity inside PV baffle opacity is the SVC-IVC baffle opening into the left ventricle.

Case study: MA # 196

Patient a baby boy, was first seen at 50-days of age with diagnosis of a large membranous VSD (ventricular septal defect). After 2 1/2 months of age his hyperkinetic pulmonary hypertension did not respond to therapy. A CT angio was performed to rule out pathology contributing to pulmonary hypertension. As there was no associated culprit lesion, pulmonary artery banding was recommended. As noted at one year of age PA (pulmonary artery) bifurcation stenosis, a tough iatrogenic complication of PA band migration must be tackled with at the time of total correction.

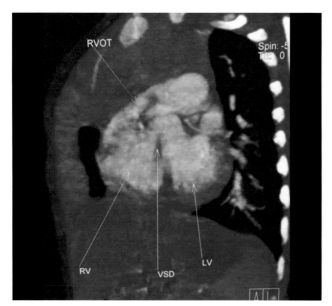 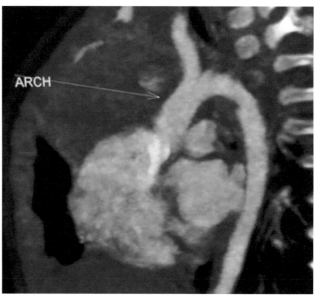

Figure 273: Large membranous VSD, with biventricular hypertrophy and normal aorta.The aortic arch is normal.There is no PDA,no CoA.

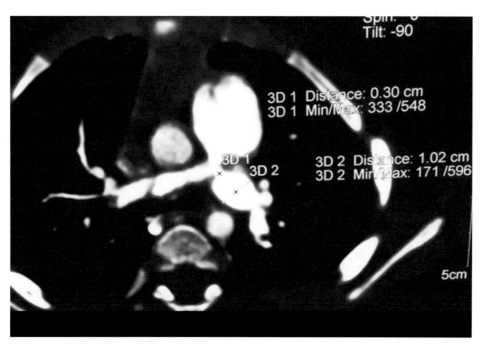

Figure 274: CT angio at one year of age, shows a tight PA band, which migrated distally to MPA bifurcation.MPA anueurysmal 1.56x in diameter,

LPA,RPA origin stenosis. RPA 0.65 cm, LPA 1.02 cm in diameter .

Case study: FM # 197

Patient a 7-year-old male,with mental motor retardation and elfine facies,was referred for a heart murmur. He had gross LVH(left ventricular hypertrophy) on EKG and chest-Xray. Echocardiography established a diagnosis of discrete subaortic stenosis with Doppler-derived peak systolic gradient of ≥ 52 mmHg.

CT angio showed the subaortic obstructive membrane, on the pre-operative study.

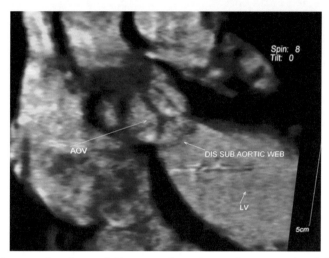

Figure 275: Note aortic valve and discrete subaortic membrane causing left ventricular outflow tract obstruction.

Case study: MS: # 189

Although rarely needed, the CT angio could be used to show an ASD. Usually clinical finding, EKG and X-Ray of the chest and echocardiography are adequate to establish the diagnosis of ASD. This particular patient was referred for the first time at the age of 7 years for a heart murmur. She was diagnosed to have ASD. She had no associated anomalies and her ASD was a secundum type defect with large left-to-right shunt.

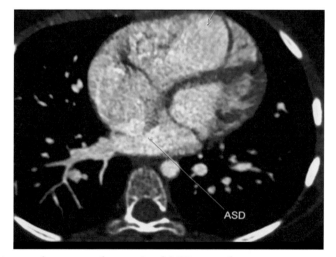

Figure 276: Arrow shows a moderate-sized ASD secundum type.

Case study: DA # 203

Patient was first seen at the age of 11 months for cyanosis and heart failure. He was found to have Ivemark syndrome, ie situs ambiguus, levocardia, with a common atrium and common ventricle,ie cor biloculare with d-TGV and severe PS (pulmonary stenosis). He had one AV (atrioventricular) valve with moderte regurgitation.At the age of 19 months he underwent AV valve repair and bilateral Glenn,ie RSVC and LSVC were implanted on the RPA and LPA respectively.He had severe PS and sub-PS, so it was decided to leave the pulmonary artery alone.

He had a stormy postoperative period. Heart failure and severe AVV (atrioventricular valve regurgitation) persisted and eventually at the age of 3 years he had a #29 metallic St-Jude valve implanted.

His improvement was remarkable. By 3 7/12 yrs of age he was fully active and his NT-proBNP was 203 pg/ml, almost within normal limits for age.

He was followed with anticongestive medications and by 8 yr of age, he was fully active, his NT- proBNP was 194 pg/ml.EKG showed LVH(left ventricular hypertrophy), RAH(right atrial hypertrophy),and LAH (left atrial hypertrophy) .

Because of financial problem, father took the patient to another hospital where at 8 1/2 yrs of age he was catheterized in preparation for tunnel anastomosis. Catheterization under **general anesthesia** showed a systolic pulmonary artery pressure of 24 mmHg. Operation,ie last stage of Fontan was denied because of high PA (pulmonary artery) pressure. Patient came back to the author. Radial artery pressure at room air was 114/61mmHg (awake), 90/50 mmHg (asleep under Midazolam).Arterial blood gas study in room air showed pH 7.36, PCO2 39 mmHg, PO2 in 55 mmHg, sat 85%. Pulmonary artery pressure via the right subclavian vein through Glenn shunt varied between 14-15/1-2 mmHg,(mean 7 mmHg), to 8-11 / 2 mmHg,(mean 5 mmHg).Two weeks later a tunnel bypassing the heart was made with a fenestrum. Postoperatively EF(ejection fraction) was 67% (Simpson's rule), PS (pulmonary stenosis) peak gradient was 67 mmHg. No fenestral flow was noted. While sitting PA pressure was 18/12 (mean 15)mmHg, supine 11/6 (mean 8) mmHg.

Three weeks postop his pulse oximetry showed a saturation of 92%.

Six weeks postoperatively, he underwent EECP therapy to improve ventricular function. At 9 years of age,the patient is fully active and asymptomatic.

The following CT angio frames are from the study before the last operation, ie IVC-PA tunnel.

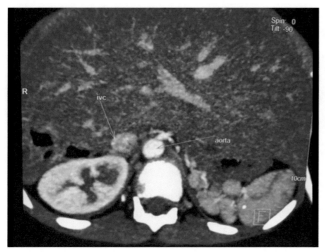

Figure 277: Midline liver, aorta and IVC side-by-side, situs ambiguus.

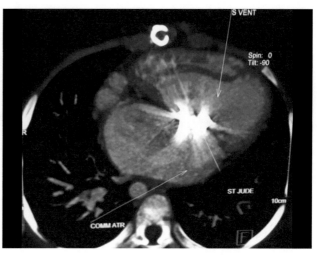

Figure 278: Levocardia, St-Jude atrioventricular valve, common atrium and single ventricle.

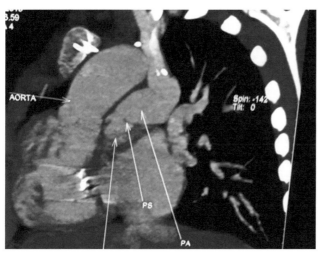

Figure 279: Common atrium, single ventricle, d-TGV, pulmonary and sub-pulmonary stenosis.

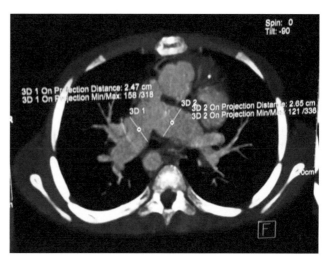

Figure 280: Confluent PA of adequate size.

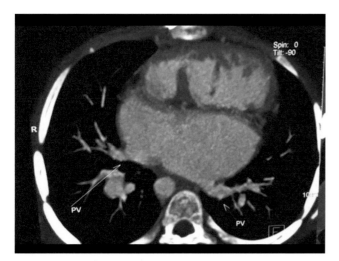

Figure 281: Pulmonary veins draining into the common atrium.

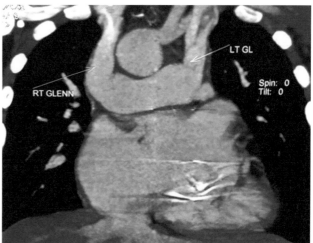

Figure 282: Right and left Glenn shunts.

Case study: AHH # 240

Patient is a 6-year-old boy, first seen at 20 months of age by a pediatric cardiologist. He had a large membranous VSD (ventricular septal defect), for which he underwent total correction at 2 years of age. He was lost to follow-up,until 5 years of age when he presented with 4 weeks history of "pneumonia" unresponsive to therapy.

He was anemic, his spleen was enlarged, and on echocardiography he had a mobile clot on the tricuspid valve. Apex of the RV (right ventricle) was full of clots and he had cough and "pneumonia" due to shower emboli.

A CT-angio was obtained and surgical removal of all the SBE-induced thrombi was recommended. The father did not follow the advice and went to his primary cardiologist who continued treating him for SBE and subsequently referred him to the surgeon to remove the infected thrombi, however at the operation no clots were found.

The pathology report of the clots removed was consistent with bacterial endocarditis. However all cultures prior to and after operation were negative. Despite negative cultures he was treated empirically with vancomycin, meropenem and gentamicin. Later on amphotericin was added to the therapeutic regimen. Because of continued fever he was switched to cephalexine and rifampin. Despite antibiotic therapy further new clots were detected on echocardiography.

Four months later he is still on antibiotics. The private physician's plan is to continue antibiotics for another four months.

Maxim: Right heart bacterial endocarditis is difficultt to diagnose and treat. Treatment with antibiotics is useless. The treatment is surgical, with <u>removal of all infected tissues.</u>

See references under bacterial endocarditis.

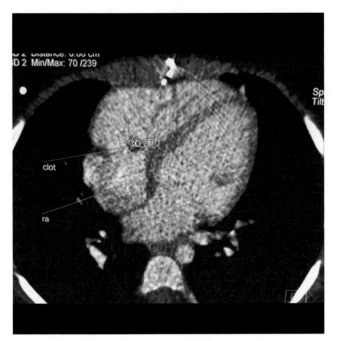

Figure 283: Clot on both sides of the VSD patch.

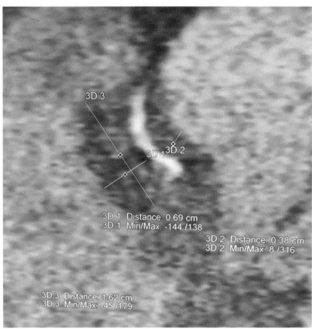

Figure 284: VSD patch with clot on both sides.

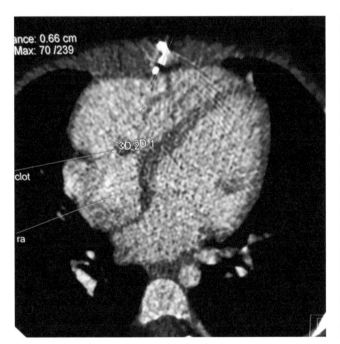

Figure 285: Clot on the tricuspid valve.

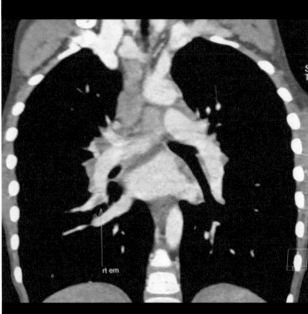

Figure 286: Pulmonary embolus (arrow).

Case study: MHK: # 249

Patient is a 54-day-old girl who was referred for a heart murmur. Patient was in overt heart failure with pulmonary hypertension.Clinical and echocardiographic study showed a spectrum of hypoplastic left heart syndrome,ie huge ASD(atrial septal defect) primum type and a small ECD (endocardial cushion defect) type VSD, hypoplastic aortic arch, small LV(left ventricle) and LA(left atrium).

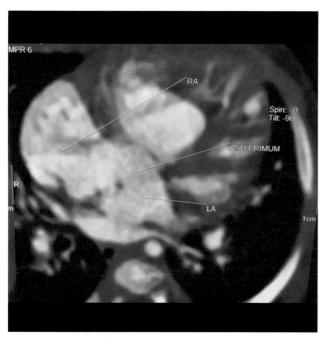

Figure 287: Huge ASD primum,large RA and RV.

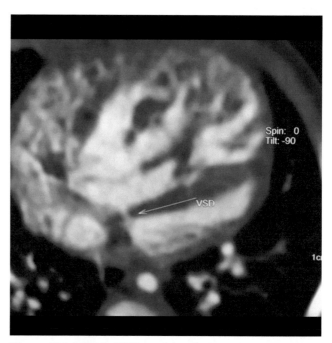

Figure 288: VSD in ECD position,huge RV,hypoplastic LV.

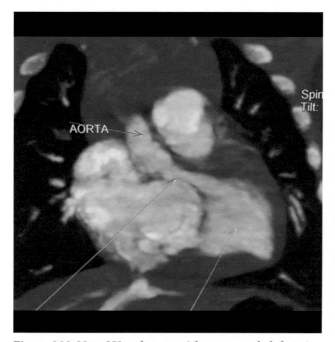

Figure 289: Note LV and aorta with goose-neck deformity of the LVOT(left ventricular outflow tract), typical of endocardial cushion defect.

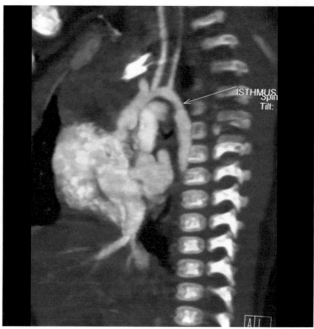

Figure 290: Hypoplastic aorta.

Case study: RSY: # 255

Patient is a 3-month-old boy with blue spells. Physical exam, EKG,chest-X-ray, and echocardiography were typical of tetralogy of Fallot.

The preop CT angio confirmed the diagnosis.

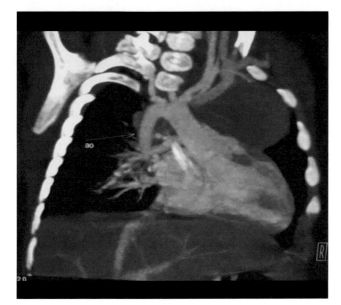

Figure 291: Right aortic arch.

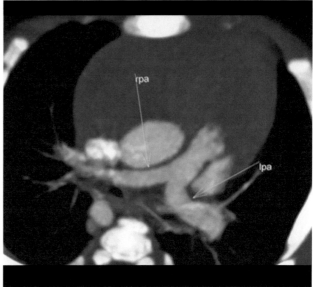

Figure 292: Confluent PA and branches of adequate size.

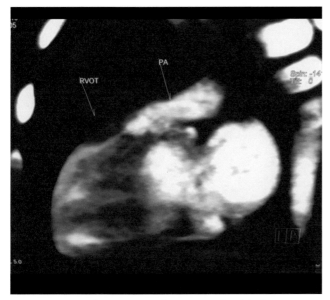

Figure 293: Tight RVOT with severe infundibular hypertrophy.

Case study: MBN: #214:

Patient is a 13-year-old male with history of congenital heart disease since at least 4 years of age. He had an operation elsewhere for VSD (ventricular septal defect) and pulmonary stenosis. Postoperatively a VVI pacemaker for complete AV block was implanted.

He had signs and symptoms of severe heart failure. Clinical and echocardiographic study revealed situs inversus with mesocardia. He had atrial fibrillation.RA(right atrium) was thus left sided and LA(left atrium) was right-sided. The RV(right ventricle) was on the right with aorta arising from it. LV(left ventricle) was on the left from which PA(pulmonary artery) arose with moderate PS (pulmonary stenosis). The tricuspid valve, supporting the systemic circulation, showed severe regurgitation.Thus patient had LTGV in situs inversus. Following CT angio he was referred to surgeon for TV replacement. However the patient expired suddenly on the way to the cardiac surgeon's office.

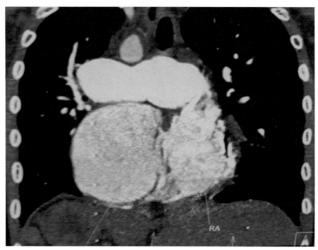

Figure 294: Situs inversus, mesocardia, Note RA on the left, LA on the right.LA is grossly enlarged due to tricuspid regitation.

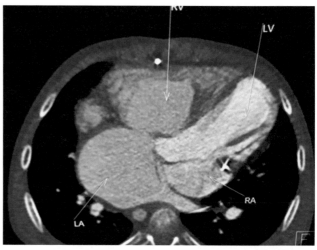

Figure 295: Corrected transposition.RV to the right, connected to the LA. LV on the right connected to the RA.

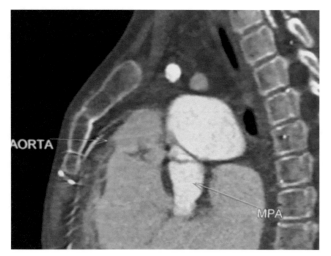

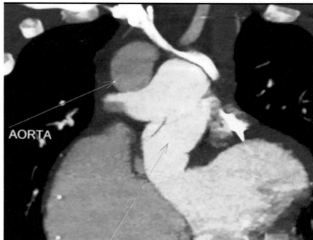

Figure 296: CTGV, MPA to the left and posterior, aorta to the right and anterior.

Case study: PN: #238

Patient a 10 year-old-male was first seen with fibromuscular subaortic aortic stenosis.Peak gradient was 44 mmHg and there was mild aortic regurgitation. Surgical correction was advised and operation was performed 2 months after the first visit. Postoperatively the gradient across the LVOT (left ventricular outflow tract) was 22 mmHg by Doppler and there was mild AR(aortic regurgitation). The patient was seen at one year intervals. At 13 1/2 years of age there was no regrowth of the subaortic tissue, however moderate MR(mitral regurgitation) was noted. LAVI (left atrial volume index) was 87 ml/m² and LVH by voltage criteria was again noted on EKG. Echocardiography showed an iatrogenic fistula between the LV(left ventricle) and the LA (left atrium) at the level of the anteromedial cusp of the mitral valve. CT angio confirmed the diagnosis. Patient underwent repair of the mitral valve and closure of the fistulous tract at 15 years of age,with remarkable improvement in clinical status.

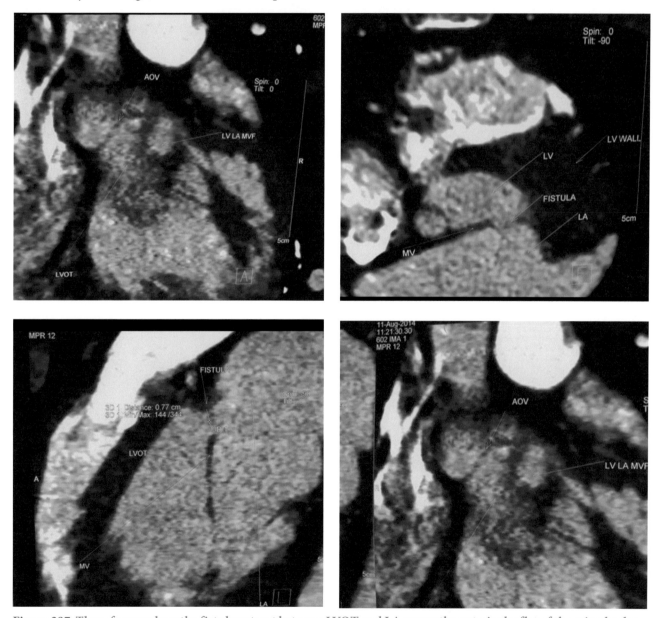

Figure 297: These frames show the fistulous tract between LVOT and LA across the anterior leaflet of the mitral valve.

Case study: AS #248

Patient is a 38 day-old-boy referred for a heart murmur. A grade 3/6 continuous murmur was present at the precordium. Chest X-ray showed gross cardiomegaly with increased pulmonary blood flow. EKG showed BVH (biventricular hypertrophy) with RVH (right ventricular hypertrophy) more remarkable than LVH (left ventricular hypertrophy). ST-segments were depressed and T waves were negative in V4R-V4, showing gross biventricular ischemia. (See below.) Echocardiography showed a small PDA (patent ductus arteriosus), a moderate-sized ASD (atrial septal defect) secundum type. The LCA (left coronary artery) was normal, however the RCA (right coronary artery) ostium was large. RCA proper was anuerysmal and opened into the high RA (right atrium).

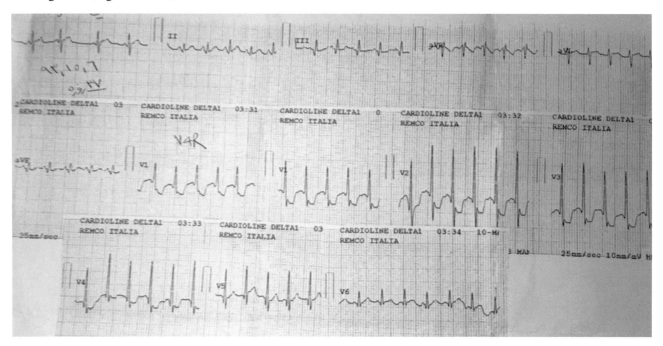

A CT angio was performed.

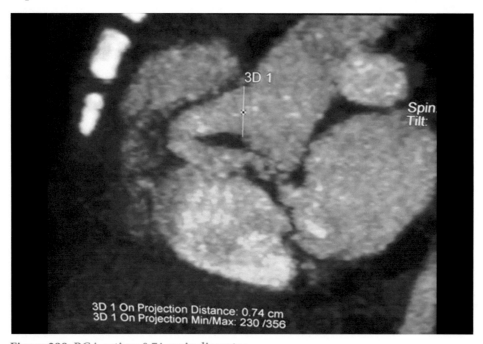

Figure 298: RCA ostium 0.74 cm in diameter.

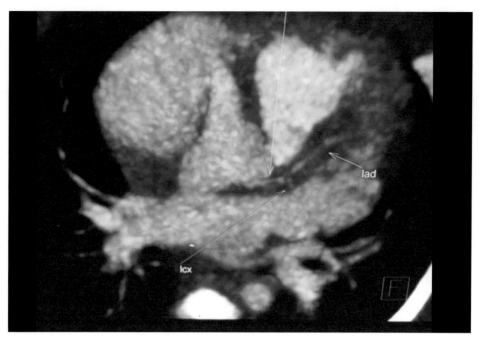

Figure 299: LCX,left main and LAD coronary arteries are normal.

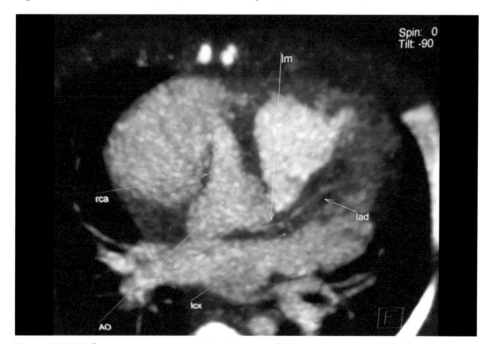

Figure 300: Left coronary artery system is normal. Note aneurysmal RCA.

CHAPTER 5

REFERENCES

In The Internet and Computer Age it is easy to add a few hundred cosmetic references to any work, however the authors would rather limit the references for this work to a limited and very pertinent articles.

Note: References are alphabetically arranged according to the topic. No reference numbers are given in the text.

Aortic valve: aortic regurgitation and aortic stenosis.

Farasat SM. Bicuspid aortic valve disease beyond the aortic root. J Am Coll Cardiol 2010; 55:699-670.
Siu SC, Silverside CK. Bicuspid aortic valve disease. J Am Coll Cardiol 2010; 55:2789-2800.
Cruz-Castaneda B, Carillo-Llamas F, Ramos-Higuera S, et al. Surgical repair of supravalvular aortic stenosis with use of Brom's technique.Tex Heart Inst J 2009;36:226-229.

Bacterial endocarditis:

Jiang SJ, Li BJ,Zhang T et al. Surgical treatment of isolated right-sided infective endocarditis. The Texas Heart Inst J 2011;38:639-642.
Pettersson GB.Surgical treatment of endocarditis. The Texas Heart Inst J 2011;38:667-668.

Bioprosthesis:

Carpentier A.Hemodynamic factors affecting the fate of valvular bioprosthesis. Circulation.2010;121:2083-2084.

Flameng W, Herregods MC, Vercalsteren M, et al.Prosthesis-patient mismatch predicts structural valve degeneration in bioprosthesis heart valves. Circulation.2010;121:2123-2129.

Cardiac Malpositions:

Richard van Praagh, Paul M.Weinberg, Samuel D.Smith,Ronald B.Foran, and stella Van Praagh. Chapter 26. Malpositions of the heart. pp 530-580. in

Heart Disease in Infants, Children, and Adolescents. edited by: Forest H.Adams. George C.Emmanouilides,Thomas A. Riemenschneider 4th edition.Williams and Wilkins.Baltimore,Maryland. 1983.

Milton H.Paul. Chapter 19.Complete transposition of the great arteries. pp 371-423.in Heart Disease in Infants, Children, and Adolescents. edited by: Forest H.Adams. George C.Emmanouilides,Thomas A. Riemenschneider 4th edition.Williams and Wilkins.Baltimore,Maryland. 1983.

Herbert D.Ruttenberg .Chapter 20. Corrected transposition of the great arteries. pp.424-442. in Heart Disease in Infants, Children, and Adolescents. edited by: Forest H.Adams. George C.Emmanouilides,Thomas A. Riemenschneider 4th edition.Williams and Wilkins.Baltimore,Maryland. 1983.

Sapire DW,Ho SY, Anderson RH,Rigby ML. Diagnosis and significance of atrial isomerism. Am J Cardiol 1986;58:342-346.

Coarctation of the aorta:

Brown ML,Burkhart HM, Connoly HM et al.Coarctation of the aorta. Lifelong surveillance is mandatory following surgical repair. J Am Coll Cardiol 2013;62:1020-1025.

Nielsen JC,Powell AJ, Gauvreau K, et al. Magnetic resonance imaging predictors of coarctation severity. Circulation.2005;111:622-628.

Mohiaddin R, Kilner PJ, Rees S, Longmore DB. Magnetic resonance volume flow and jet velocity mapping in aortic coarctation. J Am Coll Cardiol 1993;22:1515-1521.

Oshinski JN, Parks WJ, Markou CP, et al. Improved measurement of pressure gradients in aortic coarctation by magnetic resonance imaging. J Am Coll Cardiol 1996;28:1818-1826.

Forbes TJ, Kim DW,Du W, et al. Comparison of surgical,stent, and balloon angioplasty treatment of native coarctation of the aorta. J Am Coll Cardiol 2011;2662-2663-2674

Baumgartner H, Schima H, Tulzer G,Kühn P. Effect of stenosis geometry on the Doppler-catheter gradient relation in vitro:A manifestation of pressure recovery. J Am Coll Cardiol 1993;21:1018-1025.

CORONARY ARTERIES:

Angelini P. Coronary artery anomalies.An entity in search of identity. Circulation.2007; 115:1296-1305.

El-Hamamsy I, Ibrahim M, Yacoub MH.30-year outcome of anatomic correction of anomalous origin of the left coronary artery from the pulmonary artery. J Am Coll Cardiol 2011; 57:861.

Muralidaran A,Mainwaring RD,Reddy VM and Hanley FL. Prevalence of anomalous coronary arteries in pulmonary atresia with ventricular septal defect and major aortopulmonary collaterals. J Am Coll Cardiol 2013;62:1127-1128.

Maroules CD,Adams DZ,Antevil JL, et al.Anomalous origine of the right coronary artery from the pulmonary artery. The Texas Heart Inst J 2013;40:106-108.

Corrected transposition of the great vessels.(CTGV)

Mongeon FP,Connolly HM, Derani JA,et al. Congenitally corrected transposition of the great arteries. Ventricular function at the time of systemic atrioventricular valve replacemenmt predicts long-term ventricular function. J Am Coll Cardiol 2011; 57:2008-2017.

Double outlet right ventricle (DORV):

Konstantinov IE. Taussig-Bing anomaly:from original description to the current era. Tex Heart Inst J 2009;36:580-585.

Fontan operation:

Rogers LS, Glatz AC,Ravishankar C, et al. 18 years of the Fontan operation at a single institution. J Am Coll Cardiol 2012; 60:1018-1026.

Atz AM,Travison TG, McCrindle BW,et al. Late status of Fontan patients with persistent surgical fenestration. J Am Coll Cardiol 2011; 57:2437-2443.

Kawazaki disease

Gordon JB,Kahn AM,Burns JC. When children with Kawasaki disease grow up. J Am Coll Cardiol 2009; 54:1911-1920.

Gersony WM.The adult after Kawasaki disease. The risk for late coronary events. J Am Coll Cardiol 2009; 54:1921-1923.

McCrindle BW. Kawazaki disease. A chilhood disease with important consequences into adulthood. Circulation.2009;120:6-8.

Kitamura S,Tsuda E, Kobayashi J,et al:Twenty-five-year outcome of pediatric coronary artery bypass surgery for Kawazaki disease. Circulation.2009;120:60-68.

Tierney ES,Gal D,Gauvreau K, et al.Vascular health in Kawasaki Disease. J Am Coll Cardiol 2013;62:1114-1121.

NT-proBNP:

Law YM, Hoyer AW, Reller MD et al. Accuracy of plasma- B-type natriuretic peptide to diagnose significant cardiovascular disease. J Am Coll Cardiol 2009; 54:1467-1475.

Socrates T, Arenja N,Mueller C. B-type natriuretic peptide in children. J Am Coll Cardiol 2009; 54:1476-1477.

Eindhoven JA, van den Bosch AE, Ruys TP, et al.N-Terminal pro-B type natriuretic peptide and its relationship with cardiac function in adults with congenital heart disease. J Am Coll Cardiol 2013;62:1203-1212.

Eindhoven JA,vav den Bosch AE,Jansen PR, et al.The usefulness of brain natriuretic peptide in complex congenital heart disease. J Am Coll Cardiol 2012;60:2140-2149.

Pulmonary arteries:

Muraalidaran,M,Mainwaring PD,Reddy VM,et al.: Prevalence of anomalous coronary arteries in pulmonary atresia with ventricular septal defect and major aortopulmonary collaterals. J Am Coll Cardiol 2013;62:1127-1128.

Radiation dose:

Ref.Link:RadiationEmittingProductsandProcedures/Medicalimaging/MedicalXRays/ucm115332.htm Radiation quantities and units.

Hausleiter J,Meyer T, Hermann F et al. Estimated radiation dose associated with cardiac CT angiography. JAMA 2009;301(5):500-507.

Raff GL,Chinnaiyan KV,Share DA et al. Radiation dose from cardiac computed tomography before and after implementation of radiation dose-reduction techniques. JAMA 2009;301(22) 2340-2348.

Perisinakis K,Seimenis I,Tzedakis A, et al. Individualized assessment of radiation dose in patients undergoing coronary computed tomographic angiography with 256-slice scanning. Circulation.2010;122:2394-2402.

Scimitar syndrome:

Vida VL, Padalino. MA, Boccuzzo G, et al. Scimitar Syndrome. Circulation. 2010;122:1159-1166.

Total or partial anomalous pulmonary venous drainage (TAPVD;PAPVD):

Seale AN,Uemura H, Ho SY, et al: Total anomalous pulmonary venous connection. Morphology and outcome from an international population-based study. Circulation.2010;122-2718-2726.

Tetralogy of Fallot:

Lee C,Kim YM, Lee CH et al. Outcomes of pulmonary valve replacement in 170 patients with chronic pulmonary regurgitation after relief of right ventricular outflow obstruction. J Am Coll Cardiol 2012;60:1005-1014.

Bove T,Bouchez S, De Hert S et al.Acute and chronic effects of dysfunction of right ventricular outflow tract components on right ventricular performance in a porcine model. J Am Coll Cardiol 2012; 60:64-71

Cavalcanti PEF, Sá MPBOJ;Santos CA, et al.Pulmonary valve replacement after operative repair of tetralogy of Fallot. J Am Coll Cardiol 2013;62:2227-2243.

Villafañe J, Feinstein JA, Jenkins KJ, et al.: Hot topics in tetralogy of Fallot. J Am Coll Cardiol 2013;62:2155-2166.

Frigiola A, Tsang V, Bull C, et al. Biventricular response after pulmonary valve replacement for right ventricular outflow tract dysfunction. Is age a predictor of outcome? Circulation. 2008;118: S182-S190.

Shakibi JG, Rastan H, Nazarian I, Paydar M, Aryanpour I, Siassi B. Isolated unilateral absence of the pulmonary artery. Review of the world literature and guidelines for surgical repair. Japanese Heart Journal 19: 439-451,1978.

Transposition of the great vessels (TGV):

Anderson BR, Ciarleglio AJ,Hayes DA,et al: Earlier arterial switch operation improves outcome and reduces costs for neonates with transposition of the great arteries. J Am Coll Cardiol 2014:63:481-487.

Tobler D, Williams WG, Jegatheeswaran A, et al. Cardiac outcome in young adult survivors of the arterial switch operation for transposition of the great arteries.

J Am Coll Cardiol 2011; 56:58-64.

Tricuspid Regurgitation:

Rogers JH,Bolling SF.The tricuspid valve.Current perspective and evolving management of tricuspid regurgitation. Circulation.2009;119:2718-2725.

EPILOGUE

In this treatise we have described the superb contribution of cardiovascular CT-angiography to delineate most complex congenital heart anomalies.

The author (JGS) has been actively involved in pediatric cardiology, since 1970. Over the years he has observed several unique cases. He discussed these cases with Richard van Praagh, and the rare specimens were donated to The Department of Pathology of Boston Children's Hospital under Dr. van Praagh.

Here these rare and complex cases are discussed in detail, with the intention that all these cases could be easily diagnosed by CT angiography. Although none of these cases had CT-angio studies, because CT angio did not exist in those years, however they represent potential problems, which could serve as examples in which CT angio could marvelously depict the anatomy.

Case 1-Truncus-transposition:

This case was found by JGS while reviewing the pathology specimens at the Kansas University Medical Center, in 1971. Presented to Richard van Praagh at a conference, and finally classified as a rare anomaly ie a truncus with subtruncal conus, the so-called truncus transposition.

CHILDREN'S HOSPITAL
DEPARTMENT OF PATHOLOGY
300 LONGWOOD AVENUE
BOSTON, MA 02115
(617)735-7431

PATIENT NAME	BIRTH DATE 01/01/90	SEX M	ACCESSION # C-92-00407	MEDICAL RECORD # (0010)224190
PROCEDURE DATE 12/30/92	RECEIVED 12/30/92	LOCATION CLIE/CLIE	PHYSICIAN SHAKIBI, JAMI G.	

CONSULT PATHOLOGY REPORT

DIAGNOSIS:

Jami Shakibi, M.D., F.A.C.C.
Pediatrician and Pediatric Cardiologist
Africa (Jordan) Avenue
Morvarid 9TR
Sepidar B-22
Tehran, 19158
IRAN

Dear Jami:

Warmest best wishes to you. So wonderful to hear from you after all these years.

I will never forget the case of truncus arteriosus communis with a complete subtruncal muscular infundibulum and with the truncus arising entirely above the right ventricle that you kindly showed me many years ago. This was the first case of truncus with a complete subtruncal muscular infundibulum that I had ever seen. We show slides of your case almost every time I am asked to talk about truncus, and have referred to it in several publications, but thus far I don't think we have ever actually published the photographs. This is one of many things that I should have done and would like to do.

We are hoping to write a book based on the pathologic anatomy of more than 3000 cases, and I hope that we will be granted the time and strength to do this, and if the Fates permit I certainly want to give you credit for this fantastic case of truncus with a complete subtruncal muscular infundibulum.

Jami, you've done it again. The patient that you wrote to me about on December 18, 1992, by the name of Shirzadi Armin, who was then 2 years of age. We assume that the date of his cardiac catheterization was 3/31/91 (not 1971 - as the record inadvertently says).

In the interests of clarity and brevity, permit me to attempt to formulate an anatomic diagnosis, which must remain somewhat tentative, based on presently available data.

DIAGNOSES
Isolated levocardia
Probable polysplenia syndrome, this being suggested by the presence of an
    azygos extension going from the inferior vena cava which is left-sided in
                        ** CONTINUED **

PATIENT NAME	BIRTH DATE 01/01/90	SEX M	ACCESSION # C-92-00407	MEDICAL RECORD # (0010)224190
PROCEDURE DATE 12/30/92	RECEIVED 12/30/92	LOCATION CLIE/CLIE	PHYSICIAN SHAKIBI, JAMI G.	

CONSULT PATHOLOGY REPORT

DIAGNOSIS:

the abdomen to a right-sided superior vena cava, the possibility of polysplenia also being supported by the presence of a coronary sinus rhythm in the electrocardiogram

[I,L,S], i.e.,

Situs inversus (basically) of viscera and atria (I), with the inferior vena cava switching from the left side to the right side via an azygos extension at the level of the liver (diagnosis of situs inversus of the atria remains speculative and uncertain, because we have very little definite data concerning the hepatic veins, the presence of a left-sided superior vena cava, the connections of the pulmonary veins, the status of the atrial septum, the location of the coronary sinus ostium - if present, and the status of the atrioventricular canal) We cannot exclude the possibility of situs solitus of the atria. We do not know about the configuration of the atrial appendages. However, we think that the air bronchogram in the chest x-rays is suggestive of situs inversus of the lungs with a left-sided right mainstem bronchus and a right-sided left mainstem bronchus. Thus, we think that the azygos extension is going from the left-sided inferior vena cava into a right-sided superior vena cava, and that this right-sided superior vena cava may well be opening through an unroofed coronary sinus, i.e., a large coronary sinus septal defect into the right-sided left atrium

L-loop ventricles (L) (we think that this is very clear, based on your really excellent angiocardiograms)

Superoinferior ventricles, with ventricular septum abnormally horizontal and with right ventricular sinus abnormally superior relative to left ventricular sinus

High subaortic conoventricular type of ventricular septal defect (between the infundibuloarterial part of the heart above and the ventricular septum and septal band part of the heart below, the ventricular septal defect not being apparently very large

Solitus normally related great arteries (S), with apparent aortic right-sided mitral direct fibrous continuity and with an apparently well developed muscular subpulmonary infundibulum with no pulmonary-atrioventricular fibrous continuity

Undyed blood entering from the right-sided atrium illuminates the interior of the right-sided atrioventricular orifice, which looks like a right-sided mitral valve, not like a common atrioventricular valve (we don't see this really well enough to be certain, but this is our present best impression)

** CONTINUED **

FINAL REPORT INSERT INTO MEDICAL RECORD	REPORT DATE AND TIME: 05/04/93 1537 PAGE #: 2

CHILDREN'S HOSPITAL
DEPARTMENT OF PATHOLOGY
300 LONGWOOD AVENUE
BOSTON, MA   02115
(617)735-7431

PATIENT NAME	BIRTH DATE	SEX	ACCESSION #	MEDICAL RECORD #
	01/01/90	M	C-92-00407	(0010)224190

PROCEDURE DATE	RECEIVED	LOCATION	PHYSICIAN
12/30/92	12/30/92	CLIE/CLIE	SHARIBI, JAMI G.

CONSULT PATHOLOGY REPORT

DIAGNOSIS:

SUMMARY: Briefly, this appears to be the polysplenia syndrome with isolated levocardia, interruption of the inferior vena cava, azygos extension from a left-sided inferior vena cava to a right-sided superior vena cava, with the very rare and perhaps previously unknown or unpublished segmental situs set of [I,L,S], with subaortic conoventricular type of ventricular septal defect, and a patent ductus arteriosus.

In words, this appears to be isolated infundibuloarterial noninversion [A{I},L,S].

The probability of situs ambiguus is indicated by the symbol {A}, but with the impression that the atrial situs is basically situs inversus being indicated by the symbol {I}.

Jami, if we are right, this is isolated infundibuloarterial noninversion in the sense that the other two main parts of the heart - the atria and the ventricles - are inverted, whereas the infundibulum and the great arterial part of the heart are not inverted.

If upon careful two-dimensional echocardiographic or even angiocardiographic assessment it turns out that the atrial situs is in fact in situs solitus, this would then be the more familiar [S,L,S], or briefly in words, isolated ventricular inversion, again the atria and the infundibuloarterial part of the heart being noninverted.

Assuming that this is basically isolated infundibuloarterial noninversion [I,L,S], this is - to the best of my present knowledge - a previously undescribed form of congenital heart disease, i.e., a "new" entity that would be the mirror-image of isolated infundibuloarterial inversion [S,D,I] we published in 1988 in the American Heart Journal, volume 116:1337-1350, 1988, in which the first author was Dr. Ronald B. Foran.

Since that time, we have been looking for this entity which I think you may very well have beautifully represented in this case.

In terms of segmental alignments and connections, again assuming that this is [I,L,S], it is noteworthy that there is atrioventricular concordance and that there is also ventriculoarterial concordance. In other words, the segmental set itself is no reason for the patient's cyanosis and elevation of hematocrit. We think that there is an abnormal communication between the right-sided superior vena cava and the right-sided morphologically left
** CONTINUED **

175

CHILDREN'S HOSPITAL
DEPARTMENT OF PATHOLOGY
300 LONGWOOD AVENUE
BOSTON, MA 02115
(617)735-7431

PATIENT NAME	BIRTH DATE	SEX	ACCESSION #	MEDICAL RECORD #
	01/01/90	M	C-92-00407	(0010)224190
PROCEDURE DATE	RECEIVED	LOCATION	PHYSICIAN	
12/30/92	12/30/92	CLIE/CLIE	SHAKIBI, JAMI G.	

CONSULT PATHOLOGY REPORT

DIAGNOSIS:

atrium. Consequently, systemic venous blood is returning to the right-sided atrium and then enters the right-sided morphologically left ventricle and then is ejected into the aorta which originates from this right-sided LV.

If we are right about the diagnosis, this means that the patient's desaturation and cyanosis could be corrected by directing all of the systemic venous return into the left-sided atrium and thence via the left-sided right ventricle into the pulmonary artery.

Conversely, all of the pulmonary venous return should be directed, of course, to the right-sided left ventricle and thence to the aorta. The ventricular septal defect should also be closed in order to avoid the development of pulmonary vascular obstructive disease which could make this patient inoperable.

In other words, again if we are right, the systemic and pulmonary venous pathways might very well need to be reconstructed at the atrial level, plus closure of the ventricular septal defect.

Even if this is the commoner [S,L,S], i.e., isolated inventricular inversion, then atrial switch operation of the Senning or Mustard type is all that is required to hemodynamically correct the systemic and pulmonary circulations. An atrial switch procedure in [S,L,S] results in a physiologic and in an anatomic repair because the aorta originates from the left ventricle and the pulmonary artery from the right ventricle.

Jami, I think this is very very interesting and exciting, from the medical scientific standpoint, because you may very well have a newly discovered entity here - something that we have been looking for for the past five years - ever since we knew that isolated infundibuloarterial inversion exists.

The proof of the fact that the infundibular and great arterial parts of this patient's heart are not inverted is provided by the fact that the main pulmonary artery is to the left of the ascending aorta. When the infundibulum and great arteries are inverted, the main pulmonary artery passes to the right of the ascending aorta.

However, the presence of atrioventricular and ventriculoarterial concordance mean that any cyanosis which the patient definitely does have is not related to segmental discordances, but rather to the aforementioned associated malformations, particularly the right-to-left shunt via an unroofed coronary

** CONTINUED **

FINAL REPORT   REPORT DATE AND TIME: 05/04/93 1537
INSERT INTO MEDICAL RECORD   PAGE #:   4

CHILDREN'S HOSPITAL
DEPARTMENT OF PATHOLOGY
300 LONGWOOD AVENUE
BOSTON, MA 02115
(617)735-7431

PATIENT NAME	BIRTH DATE	SEX	ACCESSION #	MEDICAL RECORD #
	01/01/90	M	C-92-00407	(0010)224190
PROCEDURE DATE	RECEIVED	LOCATION	PHYSICIAN	
12/30/92	12/30/92	CLIE/CLIE	SHAKIBI, JAMI G.	

CONSULT PATHOLOGY REPORT

DIAGNOSIS:

sinus into the left atrium (as above).

SUGGESTED PLAN OF ACTION: Jami, you and your colleagues may very well already have done this, but we all think that it is important to clarify the anatomic status of the patient's atrial segment. Specifically, where do the hepatic veins drain, or if you wish, into which atrium is the suprahepatic segment of the inferior vena cava connected?

What about the state of the atrial septum?

Is there a left superior vena cava?

What is the status of the pulmonary veins?

What is the configuration of the atrial appendages?

Is it possible to ascertain the state of the spleen in this case (any evidence of the splenic artery angiocardiographically, etc)?

In other words, it is crucially important to establish whether or not the atria are basically in situs inversus, or basically in situs solitus.

Also in 1988, we published a paper concerning the echocardiographic and anatomic findings in atrioventricular discordance with ventriculoarterial concordance (Am J Cardiol 1988; 62:1256-1262).

It turns out that of the 6 predictable anatomic types of atrioventricular discordance with ventriculoarterial concordance, 5 of the 6 have been described. At that time, only [I,D,I] had not been documented. As you know, the commonest form of atrioventricular discordance with ventriculoarterial concordance is isolated ventricular inversion [S,L,S], which was present in 14 of our 25 cases. In all types of atrioventricular discordance with ventriculoarterial concordance, an atrial switch operation of the Senning or Mustard type is indicated in order to produce both the physiologic and an anatomic repair. This could be the situation in your patient, no matter what the diagnosis of the atrial situs is, if there is a sizeable coronary sinus septal defect or unroofing of the coronary sinus which permits the systemic venous return to flow into the left ventricle and thence out the aorta.

Jami, please do let me know what your thoughts are concerning the atrial situs.

** CONTINUED **

FINAL REPORT
INSERT INTO MEDICAL RECORD

REPORT DATE AND TIME: 05/04/93 1537
PAGE #:   5

CHILDREN'S HOSPITAL
DEPARTMENT OF PATHOLOGY
300 LONGWOOD AVENUE
BOSTON, MA 02115
(617)735-7431

PATIENT NAME	BIRTH DATE	SEX	ACCESSION #	MEDICAL RECORD #
	01/01/90	M	C-92-00407	(0010)224190

PROCEDURE DATE	RECEIVED	LOCATION	PHYSICIAN
12/30/92	12/30/92	CLIE/CLIE	SHAKIBI, JAMI G.

CONSULT PATHOLOGY REPORT

DIAGNOSIS:

If you and your colleagues conclude that the atria really are basically in situs inversus, then this patient has a newly discovered form of congenital heart disease which we here all think should be written up in the medical literature. We would be honored to assist in such a project, if future delineation of the anatomic status of this patient's atria, systemic veins, pulmonary veins, and atrial appendages, etc, all indicate that the patient does indeed have basically situs inversus of the atria.

If your future delineation of the atrial segment establishes that situs solitus of the atria is present, then I think that this is sufficiently well known and well documented and well established now that one would not necessarily have to publish it. However, it is a very interesting and relatively rare entity which you and your colleagues might like to publish in one of your own journals.

So Jamie, we would be honored to try to assist you, as above. Please let me know what your conclusions are and of course, if you think that the atria really are basically in situs inversus, we would very much like to see the primary data (two-dimensional echocardiography, angiocardiography, etc).

Many many thanks for being so kind as to permit us to see this fascinating case, which is potentially very exciting and perhaps may represent a newly discovered form of congenital heart disease.

Looking forward to hearing from you further about this.

With every good wish,

Most sincerely,

Richard Van Praagh, M.D.

P.S.: Just as you said in your letter, we shall retain the various things which you sent to us here, until we hear from you further. For example, I am sure we would be able to get good prints and slides of the angios from your 35 mm cineangiocardiogram. We could also make a figure of the patient's ECG.

** CONTINUED **

FINAL REPORT
INSERT INTO MEDICAL RECORD

REPORT DATE AND TIME: 05/04/93 1537
PAGE #:   6

PATIENT NAME	BIRTH DATE 01/01/90	SEX M	ACCESSION # C-92-00407	MEDICAL RECORD # (0010)224190
PROCEDURE DATE 12/30/92	RECEIVED 12/30/92	LOCATION CLIE/CLIE	PHYSICIAN SHAKIBI, JAMI G.	

CONSULT PATHOLOGY REPORT

DIAGNOSIS:
       Again, my sincerest thanks and very best wishes.

              RICHARD VAN PRAAGH, MD, DIRECTOR, CARDIAC REGISTRY 05/04/93
              (electronic signature)

MATERIALS RECEIVED:
       X-ray, angiogram

GROSS DESCRIPTION:
       None given

              RICHARD VAN PRAAGH, MD   /gg 04/27/93

                          ** END OF REPORT **

Further comments about the two new entities documented above:

Case 1-Truncus arteriosus with subtruncal conus:

As noted before left ventricle (LV) has no subarterial conus, whereas right ventricle (RV) is anatomically distinguished from LV by having a subpulmonary conus. Embryologically however when the ventricles are developing under the truncus arteriosus, vestiges of two conuses are present. However the subpulmonary conus develops as a distinct anatomical component of the right ventricle, interposed between the main pulmonary artery (MPA) and the right ventricular body. On the left however aorta is directly connected to the LV, there being no subaortic conus.

In transposition of the great arteries, aorta arises above the RV, with conus in between. On the left side, however MPA originates from the LV without an interposed conus.

In the very rare case described above by the author (JGS, in 1971 Kansas University Medical Center, Kansas City,Kansas) the very rare thing has happened,.ie truncus arteriosus was present with an interposed subtruncal conus. In truncus however there is almost never a conus present. Embryologically it can be speculated that the conus arteriosus under the aortic valve has grown, pushing the truncus upwards. Theoretically both arterial trunks could have a conus underneath. However the conus on the LV side almost never grows.

Case 2- S.A.

Isolated infundibular inversion:

2-Isolated infundibular inversion:See Dr Van Praagh's letter.Page 4, paragraph 6.

JAMI G SHAKIBI, M D, FACC.

Pediatrician

Pediatric Cardiologist

Lab — 655443
Phone: Hospital — 291010
Residence — 293454

دکتر جامی شکیمی گیلانی

پزشک ویژه ی بیماریهای کودکان و دل کودکان

آزمایشگاه ۶۵۵۴۴۲

بیمارستان ۲۹۱۰۱۰

خانه ۲۹۳۴۵۴

May,17,1993

Dr.Richard Van Praagh
Cardiac Registry
Children's Hospital
300 Longwood Ave.
Boston,MA 02115

Dear Dick:

It was indeed a most pleasant surprise to receive your kind letter and the comprehensive report dated 5/5/ 93.
Dick after so many years the memory of your superb personality and outstanding teaching is cherished by this pupil of yours.Let me tell you that

The case of Shirzadi,Armin was one of these,however as far as I know that patient must be still alive.We do not have an autopsy on him.As regards to your questions and suggestions:

    1-I do not have any further data in my hands at this moment.Therefore the bulk of the information is in you good hands.

    2-I shall do my best to locate the patient's file and see whether or not I could collect any further information.I may even try to find the pt's address and call him back to the hospital.

    3-I and my colleagues do not have the means and knowledge to publish this case.

Once again thanks a million for your kind remarks and the very informative description of the case ,which I have already read twice,many more times to come.....!

With best wishes and warmest personal regards.

Jami G.Shakibi,MD,FACC

APRICA AVE.,MORVARID
B - 22, TEHRAN, 19158, IRAN

نشانی: خیابان آفریقا ـ کوچه مروارید
ب ۲۲ ـ تهران ۱۹۱۵۸ ایران

Below see my drawing of the patient's heart on the 2nd page of Dr Van Praagh's letter.

DEPARTMENT OF PATHOLOGY
300 LONGWOOD AVENUE
BOSTON, MA 02115
(617)735-7431

PATIENT NAME				
	BIRTH DATE 01/01/90	SEX M	ACCESSION # C-92-00407	MEDICA (0010).
PROCEDURE DATE 12/30/92	RECEIVED 12/30/92	LOCATION CLIE/CLIE	PHYSICIAN SHAKIBI, JAMI G.	

CONSULT PATHOLOGY REPORT

DIAGNOSIS:

the abdomen to a right-sided superior vena cava, the possibili polysplenia also being supported by the presence of a coronary rhythm in the electrocardiogram
[I,L,S], i.e.,
Situs inversus (basically) of viscera and atria (I), with the i
vena cava switching from the left side to the right side vi
extension at the level of the liver (diagnosis of situs inv
the atria remains speculative and uncertain, because we hav
little definite data concerning the hepatic veins, the pres
left-sided superior vena cava, the connections of the pulmo:
the status of the atrial septum, the location of the corona:
ostium - if present, and the status of the atrioventricular
We cannot exclude the possibility of situs solitus of the at
do not know about the configuration of the atrial appendi
However, we think that the air bronchogram in the chest
suggestive of situs inversus of the lungs with a left-si
mainstem bronchus and a right-sided left mainstem bronch
we think that the azygos extension is going from the lef
inferior vena cava into a right-sided superior vena cava
this right-sided superior vena cava may well be opening
unroofed coronary sinus, i.e., a large coronary sinus se
defect into the right-sided left atrium
L-loop ventricles (L) (we think that this is very clear, based or
really excellent angiocardiograms)
Superoinferior ventricles, with ventricular septum abnormally hor
and with right ventricular sinus abnormally superior relative
ventricular sinus

Answers to Dr Van Praagh's questions:

JAMI G. SHAKIBI, M D, FACC.

Pediatrician

Pediatric Cardiologist

Lab — 655443
Phone: Hospital — 291010
Residence — 293454

دکتر جامی شکیبی گیلانی

سکته ویژه ی بیماریهای کودکان و دل کودکان

آزمایشگاه ۶۵۵۴۴۳
بیمارستان ۲۹۱۰۱۰
خانه ۲۹۳۴۵۴

May 23 1993

Dr.Rihcard VanPraagh
Children's Hospital
Department of Pathology
300 Longwood Ave
Boston,MA.02115

Re:Shirzadi,Armin
Med Record #(0010)224190
Accession #:C-92-00407

Dear Dick:

Greetings to you.As I promised in my previous letter I got hold of
       (not an easy task.)Here are the answers to your questions(Plan
of action,your page #5):
1-The hepatic veins drain into the left-sided RA.
2-The liver is on the left side,not midline.
3-The atrial septum seems to be intact.
4-We could not show a left SVC.
5-The pulmonary veins drain into the right-sided LA.
6-We cannot idtentify the atrial appendages.(We don't have a TE probe.)
7-There is apparently one right-sided spleen.

I am enclosing a chest XR,abdominal sonographic frames,our echocardiograms
and an EKG(dated Aug.1992) for your further examination.A few notes regarding
these data.Please note that we have identified the structures as we went along
step by step.Therefore the markings on the frames are not final on the initial
frames.
1- Frame 1,shows interatrial septum(IAS).
2-Frames 2&3 show IAS,IVS(ventricular septum) and two ventricle.The papillary
   muscles and internal anatomy of the upper ventricle(closer to the transducer
   in the picture) is that of RV.
3-Frame #4 shows VSD plus AV valves.Mild straddling of the MV is noted.
4-Frames 5&6 show drainage of the hepatic veins into the left-sided RA.
5-Frames 7&8 show drainage of the pulmonary veins into the right-sided LA.
6-Four frames mounted on cardboard#9,show a left-sided liver and apparently
   only one right-sided spleen.
7-Frame #10 shows aortic arch and PA(long axis view,suprasternal)Right and
   left side of the picture are rever_sed.
8-When transducer is rotated to obtain the short axis of the aorta from the
   suprasternal notch,Frame #11,the aorta is seen inferior and to the left of
   the right SVC,which probably drains into the right sided LA.
9-I presume that the last frame #12 shows aorta(short axis) to the left;
   RPA inferior and to the right and the bulging junction of the azygos vein
   with the Right SVC to the right and superior.

AFRICA AVE ,MORVARID
B _ 22, TEHRAN, 19158, IRAN

JAMI G. SHAKIBI, M.D, FACC.

Pediatrician

Pediatric Cardiologist

Lab — 655443
Phone: Hospital — 291010
Residence — 293454

دکتر جامی شکیبی گیلانی

سک دیره ی بیاریهای کودکان و دل کودکان

آزمایشگاه ٦٥٥٤٤٣
بیمارستان ۲۹۱۰۱۰
خانه ۲۹۳٤٥٤

Page 2

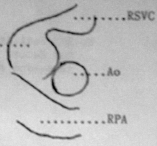

SVC-Azygos junction.... (...
(I erased the marking
here.)

......RSVC

...Ao

.........RPA

Thus your astute remark regarding an unroofed coronary sinus seems to be
correct. We were not able to detect a coronary sinus.

Credit must be given to Dr. Mohammad Mehranpour, my colleague for having performed most of the cardiac echo work-up.

Once again I would like to thank you immensely for having given your time
and attention to this case.

With best wishes and warmest personal regards.

Very Sincerely Yours.

Jami.

Jami G. Shakibi, MD.

Enc.

JGS/fa

AFRICA AVE., MORVARID
B - 22, TEHRAN, 19150, IRAN

نشانی: خیابان آفریقا ـ کوچه مروارید
ب ۲۲ ـ تهران ۱۹۱۵۸ ایران

In the following communications, after reviewing the echocardiograms chest-X-ray and angiocardiograms, the diagnosis of the entity is confirmed.

Children's Hospital
Department of Pathology

Harvard Medical School
Department of Pathology

Richard Van Praagh, M.D.

Children's Hospital
300 Longwood Avenue
Boston, MA 02115
617-735-7297

Director, Cardiac Registry
Research Associate in Cardiology
Research Associate in Cardiac Surgery

Professor of Pathology

Thursday, December 30, 1993

Jami G. Shakibi, M.D., F.A.C.C.   CONSULT#: C92-407, cont.
Pediatrician and Pediatric Cardiologist
Africa (Jordan) Avenue, Morvarid Str
Sepidar B-22
Tehran 19158
Iran

Dear Jami:

I am blushing looking a the date of your last letter to me (May 17, 1993)!

As you will no doubt recall,   may well have a previously undescribed form of congenital heart disease, namely, [I,L,S]. In words, your patient may well have situs inversus of viscera and atria, a concordant ventricular L-loop, and solitus normally related great arteries. This might be called isolated infundibuloarterial noninversion, meaning that only the infundibulum and great arteries are not inverted, whereas the ventricles, the atria and the rest of the patient have situs inversus. If this diagnosis is correct, it would be the mirror-image of [S,D,I], i.e., isolated infundibulo-arterial inversion that we described with Foran et al in 1988 (American Heart Journal 1988;116:1337-1350).

In my letter to you of May 4, 1993, in an effort to clarify the diagnosis, I had suggested the following: attempt to clarify the anatomic status of the patient's atrial segment, specifically, where do the hepatic veins drain, or to put it another way, into which atrium is the suprahepatic segment of the inferior vena cava connected?

What is the state of the atrial septum?

Is there a left superior vena cava?

What is the status of the patient's pulmonary veins?

What is the configuration of the atrial appendages?

Is it possible to ascertain the state of the spleen - any evidence of a splenic artery angiocardiographically?

Then I said that if you and your colleagues could be sure that this is situs inversus of the viscera and atria, that this patient would then indeed have the above-mentioned newly discovered form of congenital heart disease which should be written up in the medical literature. I offered to assist in this project, if the patient can be shown to have situs inversus of the atria.

On May 17, 1993, you very kindly replied and told me the following: You said that you do not have any further data at the moment.

You said that you would do your best to locate the patient's file and see whether or not you could locate any further information, and that you might be able to find the patient's address and call him back to the hospital.

You added that you and your colleagues do not have the means to publish this case and you suggested that if I wished to do so I should certainly go ahead. However, you understood that I would have to have more information concerning this patient's visceral situs, and atrial situs (as outlined in my previous letter).

Then, I received your letter dated May 23, 1993, regarding Medical Record Number (0010)224190, and our Consultation Number C92-407. You told me that the hepatic veins drain into the left-sided atrium; that the liver is on the left side, not bilaterally symmetrical; that the atrial septum seems intact; that a left superior vena cava could not be demonstrated; that the pulmonary veins drain into the right-sided left atrium; that there is one right-sided spleen; and that you could not identify or describe the morphologic characteristics of the atrial appendages, not having a transesophageal probe.

Then you guided me through the excellent echocardiographic figures that you sent to me.

These 2-D echos looked very convincing and persuasive to me. I should show them to Dr. Stephen Sanders who is the Head of our Noninvasive Laboratory here, to get his input.

Please congratulate Dr. Mohammad Mehranpour for the beautiful echocardiographic study.

So, Jami, it seems to me that the ball is very much in my court, as it were. You and your colleagues, I think, have answered the questions, very persuasively, that I raised in my earlier letter.

So now, it's up to me to find time to sit down and try and write this paper. I will then send you copies of everything for your most honest input. Please don't let me make any dumb mistakes.

So here's to a very happy new year to you and your colleagues. I am very busy, trying to write a book, as well as a flock of papers, and too many meetings. But I have never been too busy to help to write up a previously unknown form of congenital heart disease. So, congratulations, Jami!

I'll be in touch as soon as the Fates permit.

With every good wish,

Sincerely,

Richard Van Praagh, M.D.
Director, The Cardiac Registry
Research Associate in Cardiology
   and Cardiac Surgery
Children's Hospital
Professor of Pathology
Harvard Medical School
Boston, MA

P.S.: Thinking ahead to the paper, Jami, thank you very much indeed for sending me the ECG, chest x-rays, cath data, and two-dimensional echocardiography. It would be extremely helpful for us to see and to be able to photographically document the angiocardiogram that may well have been performed in this patient. To the best of my knowledge, we have never seen this patient's angio. In my letter of May 4, 1993, I wrote to you: "... we would very much like to see the primary data (two-dimensional echocardiography, angiocardiography, etc)." This is in the middle of page 6 of my consultation to you.

Jami, could you and/or your colleagues locate this patient's angiocardiograms and send them to us? We will do our utmost to get good photographs, and return the original angiocardiograms to you as soon as this has been done.

Hoping to hear from you soon, and once again – happy new year!

RVP:gg
d: 12/30/93 – t: 1/4/94

Page 2, Lines 24 25

JAMI G. SHAKIBI, M D, FACC.
Pediatrician
Pediatric Cardiologist

Lab — 655443
Phone: Hospital — 291010
Residence — 293454

دکتر جامی شکیبی گیلانی

پزشک ویژه ی بیماریهای کودکان و دل کودکان

آزمایشگاه: ۶۵۵۴۴۳
تلفن: بیمارستان: ۲۹۱۰۱۰
خانه: ۲۹۳۴۵۴

Richard Van Praagh,M.D.
Director,The Cardiac Registry
Research Associate in Cardiology and
Cardiac Surgery
Children's Hospital
Professor of Pathology
Harvard Medical School,
Boston,MA,USA

January 27,1994
Re CONSULT #:C92-407

Dear Dick:

It was indeed a great pleasure to receive your very kind letter dated December 30,1993.I wasdelighted to learn that you found the answers to your questions persuasive and above all I was elated to learn that you had kindly and magnanimously agreed to write up the case. Regarding the **angiocardiograms**,,I was quite surprised when I received them back in the mail several months ago,despite the fact that I had written to you that you may keep the angios.Referring to your letter of May 4,93,page 2 lines 24,25 and further,I presume that you have re- viewed the angiocardiograms.Probably they were copied too at the same times as the X Ray and the EKG.However if this is not the case I will send the angios to you again as soon as I find the proper means.Last

In the meantime per your suggestions delineated in your Consult C92-407 we plan to have ▆▆▆▆ operated,but because of many financial and bureau- cratic problems we have not yet been able to re-admit him to the hos- pital.Should there be any further develᶠpments I shall certainly keep you informed.
Once again thank you very much for your precious time.I also wish you

AFRICA AVE.,MORVARID
B—22, TEHRAN, 19156, IRAN

نشانی: خیابان آفریقا ـ کوچه مروارید
ب ۲۲ ـ تهران ۱۹۱۵۸ ایران

188

Children's Hospital

Monday, February 28, 1994

Jami G. Shakibi, M.D., F.A.C.C.
Pediatrician & Pediatric Cardiologist
Africa Avenue, Morvarid Street
Sepidar B-22
Tehran 19158
Iran

        Re: C92-407, cont.

Dear Jami:

Just a brief and happy word to let you know that the angiocardiograms have indeed reached me in good shape, and that I would be delighted to see you in May - any time, night or day!

I do not plan to be away in May. The only thing I have to do (apart from everything else!) is to lecture at MIT on May 16, from 10:00 AM to 12:00 noon. So I would not be at the hospital until the afternoon of May 16.

Looking forward very much indeed to seeing you, if this proves convenient and possible for you.

With every good wish.

                        Sincerely,

                        Richard Van Praagh, M.D.

RVP:gg
d: 2/28/94 - t: 3/2/94

Up to the date of publication of this book on CT angiography in congenital heart disease, I am not aware of publication of these two cases in article or book form.

The data presented here were meant to document these rare anomalies, and point out that both cases could have been easily diagnosed using CT angio.

Also see two additional new entities described in this monograph:

Case study:AA # 029 : This case shows two conuses.

Case study: HD # 081: Absence of the right ventricular sinus (apex).Spectrum of hypoplastic right heart syndrome.

ABOUT THE AUTHORS

Jami G.Shakibi,MD,FACC
Graduate of the School of Medicine, Tehran,Iran
American Board Certified in Pediatrics and Pediatric Cardiology.
Former Assistant Professor,Rush-Presbytarian St-Luke Medical Center, Chicago, Ill,USA
Former Associate Professor, Columbia University,Columbia, Mo.,USA
Former Director Pediatric Cardiology Department, and Cardiac Research Laboratory;The Cardiovascular Medical and Research Center, Tehran, Iran.
Director of Section I, Pediatric Cardiology, and director of Cardiac Research Laboratory,Day General Hospital, Tehran, Iran.

Mahmood Tehrai,MD,FSCCT, from Goa Medical College,
MD, from Mumbay School of Medicine.
Subspecialist in CT angiography and MRI.
Former assistant professor at Tehran Medical School. Tehran,Iran
Director of the Department of CT scan and MRI,Day General Hospital,Tehran,Iran

INDEX

Printed in the United States
By Bookmasters